IT HAPPENED TO ME

Series Editor: Arlene Hirschfelder

Books in the It Happened To Me series are designed for inquisitive teens digging for answers about certain illnesses, social issues, or lifestyle interests. Whether you are deep into your teen years or just entering them, these books are gold mines of up-to-date information, riveting teen views, and great visuals to help you figure out stuff. Besides special boxes highlighting singular facts, each book is enhanced with the latest reading list, websites, and an index. Perfect for browsing, there's loads of expert information by acclaimed writers to help parents, guardians, and librarians understand teen illness, tough situations, and lifestyle choices.

1. *Learning Disabilities: The Ultimate Teen Guide*, by Penny Hutchins Paquette and Cheryl Gerson Tuttle, 2003.
2. *Epilepsy: The Ultimate Teen Guide*, by Kathlyn Gay and Sean McGarrahan, 2002.
3. *Stress Relief: The Ultimate Teen Guide*, by Mark Powell, 2002.
4. *Making Sexual Decisions: The Ultimate Teen Guide*, by L. Kris Gowen, Ph.D., 2003.
5. *Asthma: The Ultimate Teen Guide*, by Penny Hutchins Paquette, 2003.
6. *Cultural Diversity: Conflicts and Challenges: The Ultimate Teen Guide*, by Kathlyn Gay, 2003.
7. *Diabetes: The Ultimate Teen Guide*, by Katherine J. Moran, 2004.
8. *When Will I Stop Hurting? Teens, Loss, and Grief: The Ultimate Teen Guide*, by Edward Myers, 2004.
9. *Volunteering: The Ultimate Teen Guide*, by Kathlyn Gay, 2004.
10. *How to Survive a Parent's Organ Transplant: The Ultimate Teen Guide*, by Tina P. Schwartz, 2005.
11. *Medications: The Ultimate Teen Guide*, by Cheryl Gerson Tuttle, 2005.

Medications

The Ultimate Teen Guide

CHERYL GERSON TUTTLE

It Happened to Me, No. 11

The Scarecrow Press, Inc.
Lanham, Maryland • Toronto • Oxford
2005

SCARECROW PRESS, INC.

Published in the United States of America
by Scarecrow Press, Inc.
A wholly owned subsidiary of The Rowman & Littlefield Publishing Group, Inc.
4501 Forbes Boulevard, Suite 200
Lanham, Maryland 20706
www.scarecrowpress.com

PO Box 317
Oxford
OX2 9RU, UK

British Library Cataloguing in Publication Information Available

Library of Congress Cataloging-in-Publication Data

Tuttle, Cheryl Gerson.
  Medications : the ultimate teen guide / Cheryl Gerson Tuttle.
      p. cm. — (It happened to me ; no. 11)
  Includes bibliographical references and index.
  ISBN 0-8108-4905-4 (hardcover : alk. paper)
  1. Teenagers—Diseases—Chemotherapy—Encyclopedias. 2. Pediatric
pharmacology—Encyclopedias. I. Title. II. Series.
RJ550.T88 2005
615.58'0835—dc22

2004011813

To Helen, Lynne, and Bob

Also to Shira for her inspiration

Disclaimer

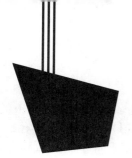

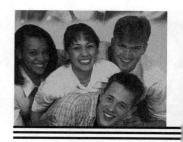

The information in this book is presented for educational purposes only. It is not intended as a substitute for medical advice but rather as a sharing of knowledge and information from the research of the author. We advise readers to seek prompt medical advice for any personal health questions. Never delay seeking medical attention because of something you have read. Your doctor or other health care professional is the best source of information related to your personal needs.

The medications listed are those most common in a particular category at the time of publication. New drugs are being tested on an ongoing basis and other drugs are gaining approval for different conditions. Some information about drugs is subject to interpretation. The author, editors, consultants, and publisher have taken great care to ensure that the information presented is accurate at the time of publication and cannot be responsible for errors, omissions, or the application of this information and the consequences arising from that application. Therefore, the author, editors, consultants, and publishers have no liability in regard to claims related to the use of the information.

It is not possible to list every brand of drug on the market for a particular condition. The brands listed are not an endorsement for that brand. They are just examples of what are available. Your doctor is the best source of the most current remedies and the best choice for you.

Not all side effects happen and it is not possible to predict how the medications will affect you. Some side effects disappear over time and some increase with continued dosages. Some of the effects can be minimized by changing when and how you take the medications. Check with your doctor or pharmacist if you are having an unusual reaction while taking a new medication. It is possible that the medication can be changed or that a slight change in the way you take it can make all the difference.

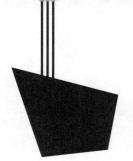

Contents

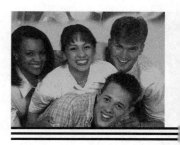

THE A TO Z GUIDE TO ILLNESSES AND DISABILITIES AND THE MEDICATIONS USED FOR THEM

Contents

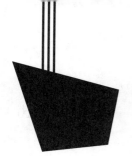

Acknowledgments

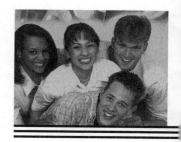

I would like to acknowledge Celia P. MacDonnell, PharmD, BS, Rph, clinical assistant professor at the University of Rhode Island College of Pharmacy, for reviewing the content of the book. Her expertise was invaluable for ensuring that the information presented conforms to what we know about medications today.

I would like to thank the many teens that contributed their voices to the chapters in this book. I promised to keep their anonymity so I will not list them by name. They know who they are. I can name and thank Dr. Michael Levine, Helen Hackwork, Kathy Glennon, and Donna Peltier-Saxe who put me in touch with the teens and showed their moral support for the process.

I would also like to thank Dr. Ronna Fried, my editor Arlene Hirschfelder, and Henry Frommer for sharing their expertise and for their friendship and support.

A special debt of gratitude goes to the many people and agencies that provided special information and graphics about how certain medications work: Alan McCord at Project Inform, Michael Ermarth and Raymond Formanek at the Federal Drug Administration, the National Institute of Allergy and Infectious Diseases, David Butler at *The Boston Globe*, Dr. Rami Burstein and Moshe Jakubowski at the Harvard Institutes of Medicine, Jennifer Allyn at the American Academy of Dermatology, Richard Silvia, PharmD at the Massachusetts College of Pharmacy and Health Sciences, Karen Leighty at the National Institute of Allergy and Infectious Diseases, and Blair Gately at the National Institute on Drug Abuse.

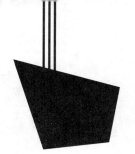

Foreword

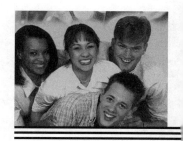

Cheryl Tuttle has taken on the daunting task of compiling an information guide to the most common medical conditions adolescents face today. In addition to this, she has assembled lists of medications commonly prescribed to treat these conditions, and done so in an easy-to-read format. She has painstakingly researched a variety of disease states and the many therapeutic choices available today.

It is our hope that this text will serve as a useful guide to enable young people to become more involved in medication decisions related to their care. To accomplish this, they must first be more informed about the choices open to them, as well as the associated benefits and risks that accompany the use of any drug.

This text is not intended to replace the advice and counsel of the health care providers treating our young people today. Rather, it is intended to provide adolescents with a baseline of knowledge related to their own drug therapy, so that they may participate more fully in their own care. Knowledge is power when used correctly.

Celia P. MacDonnell, PharmD, BS, Rph
Clinical Assistant Professor
University of Rhode Island College of Pharmacy

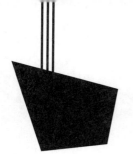

Introduction

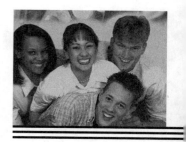

Being a teenager is hard enough without having to deal with an illness that requires medication on a regular basis. This is your time to be free to explore your interests, your limits, and your body. However, if you are reading this book, you are currently taking or contemplating taking medication for a physical or emotional problem, and that medication may place some limits on your freedom.

There are many things to deal with as a teenager. Your friends are getting their licenses to drive. In spite of the dangers, some may be involved with alcohol and drugs. Others may be dating and experimenting with sex. Sports or other physical activities may be important to your life and that of your friends. You might be staying up late studying or going to parties. Your diet probably isn't as healthy as it could be. This is also the time you begin to make plans for your career and your future. All of these things are a normal part of growing up and fitting in. Taking medications may not be seen as "normal" and it is very hard to be different at this time in your life.

The good news is that, even if you think you are the only one in this position, you are not. Most illnesses and disabilities are invisible, so you may not be aware of your friends who are also taking medications. As you read this book, you will see the large number of illnesses that require medication and I can guarantee that you know someone who has one of the conditions listed and is taking medication for it.

The other good news is that you can learn a great deal about the medication you need to take and you can use that information to help you feel in control of your situation. Your medical professionals and your parents are always a major resource for information, but adolescence is a time when you want to be more independent. Learning about your medications does not mean that you ignore your doctors or your parents. It just means that you are a contributing member to discussions about your health and you can be a part of the decisions that affect your life. You can show your independence and exert your authority with a knowledge base that shows you are an important part of your medical team.

This book is not a substitute for open and honest discussions with your doctors, nurses, pharmacists, or parents. It is not a medical text. It is one source of information about your particular illness or disability and the medications that are prescribed for that illness or disability. The most common conditions adolescents face are listed—from A to Z. The medications that are commonly used for that disease are listed and, where known, there is a description of how they work in your body. Their generic or chemical ingredients are listed and one brand name is listed after that. In many cases, there are more than one or two brands with the same generic ingredients and the brand name listed is not an endorsement for that particular brand.

Common side effects for a type of medication are listed so you will have information to know if the possible side effects are a major problem for you. Sometimes another medication without a particular side effect can be substituted. (If a side effect of your medication is drowsiness and you have an after-school job that requires you to be alert, you might ask your doctor if there is something else you can take that won't have that side effect.) Where possible, there will be information about interactions with foods and other drugs. (Some medications are not as effective or have different side effects if you are taking birth control pills, for example.) It is not possible or reasonable to list every possible side effect for a particular medication. Also, there is not clear consensus about the most common side effects. The side effects listed apply to the class of drugs (unless otherwise indicated) and include only common side effects found in at least two reliable sources that list drug information. There might be other side effects that occur to you so you should be alert to any unusual changes in your body and report them immediately to your doctor.

Medications that are used to treat particular diseases change over time as new information is discovered and new medications are given government approval for treatment of a particular condition. Also, drugs continue to be tested even after they are approved, and new tests might discover dangerous side effects that cause the manufacturer to take that drug off the market for any or all conditions. The information

HOW THE FOOD AND DRUG ADMINISTRATION (FDA) APPROVES NEW DRUGS

Under current law, all new drugs need proof that they are effective, as well as safe, before they can be approved for marketing. But it's important to realize that no drug is absolutely safe. There is always some risk of an adverse reaction. It's when the benefits outweigh the risks that the FDA considers a drug safe enough to approve.

Before any drug gets on the market today, the FDA decides—as quickly as a thorough evaluation allows—whether the studies submitted by the drug's sponsor (usually the manufacturer) show it to be safe and effective for its intended use. Here's what goes into those decisions.

- The FDA participates actively in the drug development process, seeking to provide clear standards and expectations.
- Sponsors are encouraged to meet with the FDA. At this conference, the FDA gives advice about the design of the sponsor's study plan to ensure that the trials will be acceptable.
- The FDA also provides advice in the form of guidelines on how to study particular classes of drugs and on how to submit and analyze data in a marketing application.
- The documentation required is supposed to tell the drug's whole story, including what happened during the clinical tests, how the drug is constituted—its components and composition, results of the animal studies, how the drug behaves in the body, and how it's manufactured, processed, and packaged, especially the quality controls. The FDA also requires samples of the drug and its labels.

(continued)

- Full reports of a drug's studies must be submitted so that the FDA can evaluate the data.
- The human studies also generate information that will be in the drug's professional labeling, the guidance approved by the FDA on how to use the drug. This is the package insert that accompanies a drug in all shipments to physicians and pharmacies.
- If the FDA's evaluation of studies reveals major deficiencies, substantially more work by the sponsor may be needed, ranging from performing further analyses to conducting new studies—in either case thereby extending the evaluation time and delaying approval.

The FDA has undertaken various ways to reduce drug review time, which during the past several years has averaged (median) about two years, down from about two and a half years. In the final analysis, the FDA's decision whether to approve a new drug for marketing boils down to two questions:

1. Do the results of well-controlled studies provide substantial evidence of effectiveness?
2. Do the results show the product is safe under the conditions of use in the proposed labeling? Safe, in this context, means that the benefits of the drug appear to outweigh its risks.

Once its application is approved, a drug is on the market as soon as the firm gets its production and distribution systems going.

Adapted from Dixie Farley, "Benefit Vs. Risk: How FDA Approves New Drugs." *FDA Consumer Special Report*. January 1995.

in this book is current to the time of publication, but you might need to go to one of the websites listed at the back of the book for the most current information about the medications for your condition.

You don't have to read this book from cover to cover. Look at the medications for your situation and learn all you can about them. You might also want to look at diseases your friends have to get a better understanding of what they are going through. There might be other problems that you will want to address once you know there is a medication that can help with that problem. You can have acne as well as diabetes and you might want to learn about interactions between the medications or if there are medications that will help both conditions.

Remember that knowledge is power that can be used to make you a more responsible consumer and a more cautious and thoughtful teenager. While taking medications can seem to be a burden right now, the alternatives are worse. You are lucky to be living at a time when there are medications that help with your condition. Learn what you need to know to feel comfortable with what you need to do to help yourself.

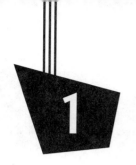

The Hows and Whys of Taking Medication

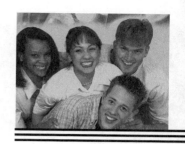

If you are reading this book, you have decided to begin to manage your own health care and to learn more about the treatments you are taking for a special medical or psychological condition. The medications you are taking are going into YOUR body so it is important that you know what they are doing to and for you. It might be easier to let your parents be in total control and make the decisions, but, at some point, you will need to be in charge of your health care and this is a good time to start. The more you learn about your condition and the treatments necessary for it, the better able you will be to adjust your lifestyle to your individual needs.

THE WHYS

Medications alone are rarely the whole answer for any condition you are facing. They are used as a part of a total treatment plan. Lifestyle changes are also important and that may be harder than taking a pill and hoping things will get better. Eating healthy; getting enough sleep; avoiding alcohol, drugs, and tobacco; and reducing stress go hand in hand with any medication regimen.

If you take medications, your doctor will determine what is best for you based on his or her expertise and experience. It is okay to question the medication you are being given, but your doctor or pharmacist is the best source you have for what works and what doesn't for the condition you have. You should ask questions. The following queries about the medications you are taking can be used as a guide in order to help you fully understand why you are taking the medications, how you should take them, and what to expect as a result:

- What are the generic and brand names of the medication?
- What is it supposed to do?
- How does it work?
- What if it doesn't work?
- How and when do I take it?
- How long will I have to take it?
- What foods, drinks, or other medications should I avoid while taking it?
- Should it be taken with food or on an empty stomach?
- Is it safe to drink alcohol while on this medication?
- Are there special precautions if this medication is combined with other medications, vitamins, or certain foods or fruit juices?
- What are the side effects, which should I report and which should I ignore?
- Are there special instructions for taking this medication?
- Are there special instructions for storing it?
- What is the expiration date? Can it be used effectively after that date?
- What do I do if I miss a dose?
- What are the signs of an overdose?
- Is there a less expensive generic brand that will work for me?

You may have heard that some of the medications available for the conditions listed have not been tested for safety in children. Your doctor may prescribe medications that have been approved for other conditions than the one you have. (For example, your doctor may prescribe a drug used for seizures to treat your migraine headache.) You may also have seen advertisements about new prescriptions drugs for your condition that sound better than what you are currently taking. This type of information can be misleading or confusing. Your doctor will know the information about the risks regarding the various medications, the current dosage to treat your condition, and the new medication long before it is advertised. You need to ask the questions, for self-knowledge, but your doctor is the best source for determining if a medication is the right one for you.

THE HOWS

When you are taking medications there are very important guidelines you must follow. The medical professionals and pharmacists must be in charge of how you take the drugs.

- Make sure you are working with medical professionals you respect and can trust. You will need to ask lots of questions and you need to be comfortable answering the questions they ask you. If confidentiality is an issue, discuss this with your doctor. Depending upon your age, your doctor may need to inform your parents of anything you disclose. You may be dealing with more than one specialist and it is important that they be able to communicate with each other also. There are some doctors who specialize in working with teens. Other specialists may see few teens and may not know how to talk to you. Be upfront if you are uncomfortable. It may not be possible to change doctors, but, at least, you can feel that your concerns are heard.

- Make sure you tell your doctor about other medical problems you have and medications you are taking. Many medications should not be used at the same time because they can increase the risk of side effects and can change the side effects you experience. Let your doctor know about over the counter products (such as cold medication or antacids) or alternative remedies you are taking. There is always the risk of adverse interaction with a particular medication and your doctor or pharmacist is the best one to tell you if what you are taking is safe. Also let your doctor know if you have allergies or if you are on a special diet. Some of the medications may contain other ingredients (like aspirin or dyes) that you might be allergic to.

- Let your doctor know if you have difficulty reading and understanding the information on the prescription label. Don't expect to keep all the instructions and precautions in your memory if you don't have the written information from the drug insert or the label to fall back on.

◎ Always take the medications in the amount prescribed. More is not always better and the dosage for you may not be the same as your friend, even if you are on the same medication for the same condition. If you think that the amount you are taking is causing unwanted side effects, discuss this with your doctor to see if there are safe adjustments you can make.

◎ Always take medications at the time and under the conditions stated by the doctor or pharmacist. This may not always be easy due to the unpredictability of your lifestyle. If you do not have meals at regular times, it may be difficult to take your medications on a "full stomach" or "empty stomach." If you do not go to sleep or wake up at regular times, this could also throw off your medication schedule. Discuss these issues with your doctor to see if there are alternatives to the schedule. If not, you will have to adjust your schedule while the medications are necessary. An alarm clock or watch might help you remember when to take your medication.

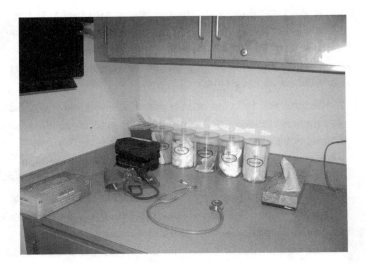

◎ Always take the medications for the number of doses prescribed. Even if you are feeling better, continue to take the medication. Some medications, particularly antibiotics, need to be taken for a full course to make sure the bacteria do not come back.

HOW TO CARE FOR YOUR PRESCRIPTIONS

Richard J. Silvia, PharmD, BCPP, Assistant Professor of Pharmacy Practice, Massachusetts College of Pharmacy and Health Sciences

Where to store them:

1. Out of children's reach or inside of a locked container that children cannot gain access to.
2. NOT near a source of heat (above a stove, appliance, baseboard, etc.) that might damage the prescription drug inside.
3. NOT near a source of moisture (near a sink, shower, etc.) that might damage the prescription drug inside.
4. NOT in direct sunlight or other bright lights since some medications are light sensitive.

*** *This means that bathroom and kitchen cupboards and shelves are NOT good storage places for medications due to the heat and moisture in kitchens and bathrooms.*
*** *High bedroom drawers or shelves out of direct sunlight and out of the reach of children make good places for medication.*

How to store them:

1. Keep the prescription in its original container as much as possible. An exception to this is if you use a pill holder to arrange your medications for the day. But only put in the medication you need for that day or week (if you own a weekly pill container).
2. Do NOT put different medications into the same container marked for a specific prescription. This could possibly cause a serious problem if you forget which medication is which.
3. If a medication needs to be refrigerated, then keep it in the fridge. Make sure it is clearly labeled as to what it is and how long it is good for. The pharmacist can help you with this.
4. If a medication is to be mixed with food before you take it, ONLY mix what you need for that immediate dose, do NOT mix up several doses in advance unless it is absolutely necessary.

Medications can affect your body in many ways—some good and some bad. You wouldn't walk onto a car lot and just buy whatever car the salesman told you to buy. You would ask questions first. Why take a medication without asking questions to understand what you are getting? Is your car worth more than your body?

- ◉ You might need a chart to help with multiple medications and multiple times when they must be taken. There is a medication diary at the end of the book. See if that works for you. You can adapt it to fit your particular condition and you can photocopy and reduce it so it will fit in your school assignment book.

- ◉ Often pills will look alike. If you are taking more than one medication, keep them in their original containers to avoid mix-ups.

- ◉ It is a good idea to fill all of your prescriptions at the same pharmacy. That way the pharmacist will have a record of everything you are taking and can be a resource for possible interactions.

- ◉ Do not substitute a generic drug for the brand name without discussing this with your doctor. Sometimes the generic drugs have subtle differences in the way they are formulated and that difference can be harmful to you and your conditions. Also, do not substitute a drug from another country or on the Web without discussing this with your doctor. These medications can have harmful side effects or can interact with other medications you are taking.

- ◉ If you are traveling, be sure to take enough medication for the time you will be away and be sure to take extra amounts to have enough to allow for any possible delays like cancelled flights or last-minute changes in your plans. If you are leaving the country, take documentation to show that your medication is a prescription for a specific condition or illness.

SIDE EFFECTS

The side effects listed in the chapters are for a class of medications rather than for particular medications in the class unless there are extreme cautions for one particular drug. All of these medicines in a class are similar, so many of the side effects may occur with any of the medicines in that class. The most common side effects are listed. There is always the possibility you might have a different side effect so be sure to check with your doctor if you experience any unusual symptoms while on these drugs.

Not everyone has side effects from medications. If you understand about side effects you will be better able to deal with them.

- Some of the side effects listed only last for a short time and go away once your body has become used to the medication. Other side effects only come after long-term use. Check with your doctor before stopping the medication due to unwanted side effects to determine what course the side effects usually take.

- When you are deciding to use a medicine, the risks of taking the medicine must be weighed against the benefit to you. Discuss this carefully with your doctor.

- Some side effects are predictable because of the way the drug works. For example, diuretics make you urinate more and this can increase the loss of sodium, potassium, and other electrolytes that are lost with the urine. Many of the side effects from this type of medication, like dry mouth, excessive thirst, and weakness, are the result of the potassium depletion. You can adjust your eating and take supplements to deal with this complication.

- The precautions about serious side effects are constantly changing and the information can be very confusing. The drug manufacturers list common side effects for their brands and websites might list different side effects for the same brand of drug. Studies done in one country may show a very dangerous side effect for a particular drug, but studies in other countries may disagree. When experts disagree, it makes it harder for you to weigh the risks of what you need to take for your condition. Use the questions above as a guideline for talking with your doctor about your concerns.

- Many of these medications can affect pregnancy and nursing. Talk with your doctor about the risks involved. Also discuss whether you can donate blood while taking certain medications since there is a possibility that it might be given to a pregnant or nursing woman.

- Many of these medications cause drowsiness, dizziness, or lightheadedness. Do not drive a car, ride a bicycle, or engage in other activities that might be dangerous until you know how the medication will affect you.

◎ You might need to take an additional medication to combat the side effects of the medication you must take. For example, if the primary medication keeps you from sleeping, you may need to take a pill designed to help you sleep. If the required medication causes severe heartburn or upset stomach, you may need another pill for that. Work closely with your doctor and pharmacist to make sure the different medications are compatible and that the combination does not cause further problems.

◎ A common concern when taking medications is that side effects are increased if you drink alcohol or use other central nervous system depressants. Central nervous system depressants other than alcohol include:

  ◎ Antihistamines and medications for allergies and colds
  ◎ Sedatives
  ◎ Sleeping medications
  ◎ Antianxiety medications
  ◎ Prescription pain medications or narcotics
  ◎ Muscle relaxants
  ◎ Anesthetics
  ◎ Medication for seizures

DRUG AND FOOD INTERACTIONS

Almost every medication has directions about how it should be taken and what should be avoided while taking it. An anxiety medication may also affect blood pressure, so you need to be careful about taking anything else that affects blood pressure. Some medications are not as effective if you take them with certain fruit juices because the acid in the juice can interact with the medication. It is not possible to list all interactions in a book of this length. Read the insert that comes from the pharmacy when you get the medication. It will tell you the basics about what you need to do and what to avoid. If the information is not clear, ask the pharmacist to explain it. Think about your lifestyle and ask the questions that are relevant to what you do and what you eat.

OVERDOSE

Many of the medications listed can have serious or life-threatening side effects if you take too much. Call your doctor immediately if you experience extreme side effects that could be a result of an overdose. If you cannot reach your doctor right away, go to the nearest hospital emergency room. Make sure you bring the pill container so medics will know what to do.

ADDICTIONS AND DEPENDENCY

Many of the medications you take can be addictive. You can keep this from happening if you are alert to the signs of addiction. You might be having a problem with the medication if you:

- Feel a strong desire or need to continue taking the medicine.
- Become obsessed with the need for more of the medication.
- Feel a need to increase the dose to receive the desired effects of the medicine.
- Self-prescribe the medication for other problems than for what it was originally intended.
- Experience withdrawal side effects (for example, mental depression, unusual behavior, or unusual tiredness or weakness) occurring after the medicine is stopped.
- Feel that you are "zonked out" or can't function well when on the medication.
- Feel "high" rather than just pain or stress free when taking medication for pain or depression.

THE BOTTOM LINE

You are now ready to check out the information about your particular illness or condition. If your doctor prescribes a medication that is not on the list, look it up by the generic ingredient on the list in the List of Medications. That way, you can learn about possible side effects and other precautions that are common to that type of medication.

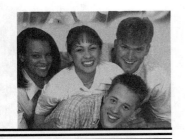

Acne

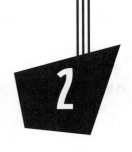

Acne is the term used for plugged pores, pimples, and deeper lumps that occur on your face, neck, and upper body. This condition usually occurs in adolescence and can be psychologically upsetting because it can be disfiguring and lead to permanent scarring.

THE MOST COMMON MEDICATIONS

Over-the-Counter (OTC) Medications

Benzoyl Peroxide (Clearasil®)

Salicylic Acid (Oxy Clean®)

Glycolic Acid (Alpha Hydroxy®)

Resorcinol (Acnomel®)

Sulfur (Cuticura®)

Prescription Topical Medications

Antibiotics

Erythromycin (Staticin®)

Clindamycin (Cleocin T-gel®)

Antibacterials

Azelaic acid lotion (Azelex®)

Benzoyl Peroxide (Clearasil Maximum Strength Medicated Anti-Acne Cream®)

> Early pioneer women treated acne with wheat water. Egyptians used honey mixed with wheat or almond oil. Catherine the Great of Russia used clay powder. The Chinese of thousands of years ago pressed on trigger points on the face and hands.
>
> Dian Dincin Buchman, *Ancient Healing Secrets: Practical Cures That Work Today* (Baltimore: Ottenheimer, 1996).

Topical Retinoids

Tretinoin (Retin-A®)

Adapalene (Differin®)

Tazarotene (Tazorac®)

Prescription Oral Antibiotics

Tetracycline (Achromycin V®)

Minocycline (Minocin®)

Doxycycline (Vibramycin®)

Erythromycin (E-mycin®)

Prescription Systemic Retinoids

Isotretinoin (Accutane®)

Prescription Hormonal Therapies

Estrogen-containing oral contraceptives (Ortho Tri-Cyclen®)

GENERAL INFORMATION ABOUT HOW THESE DRUGS WORK

The exact cause of acne is unknown, but the high hormone levels that occur at puberty may trigger it. Acne occurs when too much sebum, a semiliquid, oily substance, is produced by your glands. The sebum combines with the hair and the cells in your pores and plugs up the pores instead of emptying onto the skin. It allows bacteria, Propionibacterium acnes (P. acnes), that are normally on your skin to grow in the plugged area and sets off a chain reaction that leads to inflammation and eventually leads to pimples and other skin lumps. Lumps or lesions under the skin are called whiteheads and those above the skin are called blackheads. The acne medications interfere with this process. They do not cure acne.

MYTHS ABOUT ACNE FROM AMERICAN ACADEMY OF DERMATOLOGY

Myth #1: Acne is caused by poor hygiene. If you believe this myth, and wash your skin hard and frequently, you can actually make your acne worse. Acne is not caused by dirt or surface skin oils. Although excess oils, dead skin, and a day's accumulation of dust on the skin looks unsightly, they should not be removed by hard scrubbing. Vigorous washing and scrubbing will actually irritate the skin and make acne worse. The best approach to hygiene and acne: Gently wash your face twice a day with a mild soap, pat dry—and use an appropriate acne treatment for the acne.

Reprinted with permission from the American Academy of Dermatology, 2002. www.skincarephysicians.com/acnenet/myths.html. All rights reserved.

Acne medications work to get rid of outbreaks and prevent the forming of new ones in one or more of the following ways:

1. Reducing the production of too much sebum
2. Reducing the production of bacteria, P. acnes
3. Reducing the abnormal shedding of skin cells that clump up and block your pores
4. Reducing inflammation

OTC benzoyl peroxide kills P. acnes and may reduce oil production by drying your skin.

MYTHS ABOUT ACNE FROM AMERICAN ACADEMY OF DERMATOLOGY

Myth #2: Acne is caused by diet. Extensive scientific studies have not found a connection between diet and acne. In other words, food does not cause acne. Not chocolate. Not french fries. Not pizza. Nonetheless, some people insist that certain foods affect their acne. In that case, avoid those foods. Besides, eating a balanced diet always makes sense. However, according to the scientific evidence, if acne is being treated properly, there's no need to worry about food affecting the acne.

Reprinted with permission from the American Academy of Dermatology, 2002. www.skincarephysicians.com/acnenet/myths.html. All rights reserved.

MYTHS ABOUT ACNE FROM AMERICAN ACADEMY OF DERMATOLOGY

Myth #3: Acne is caused by stress. The ordinary stress of day-to-day living is not an important factor in acne. Severe stress that needs medical attention is sometimes treated with drugs that can cause acne as a side effect. If you think you may have acne related to a drug prescribed for stress or depression, you should consult your physician.

Reprinted with permission from the American Academy of Dermatology, 2002. www.skincarephysicians.com/acnenet/myths.html. All rights reserved.

**MYTHS ABOUT ACNE FROM
AMERICAN ACADEMY OF DERMATOLOGY**

Myth #4: Acne is just a cosmetic disease. Yes, acne does affect the way people look and is not otherwise a serious threat to a person's physical health. However, acne can result in permanent physical scars—plus, acne itself as well as its scars can affect the way people feel about themselves to the point of affecting their lives.

Salicylic acid reduces the abnormal shedding of skin cells. It helps to make the dead skin more soluble to be lifted away. It can penetrate the plugged pores and unclog them. This is found in peels and can be found in cosmetic preparations.

Salicylic acid, resorcinol, and sulfur help break down blackheads and whiteheads by attacking the bacteria.

**MYTHS ABOUT ACNE FROM
AMERICAN ACADEMY OF DERMATOLOGY**

Myth #5: You just have to let acne run its course. The truth is, acne can be cleared up. If the acne products you have tried haven't worked, consider seeing a dermatologist. With the products available today, there is no reason why someone has to endure acne or get acne scars.

Glycolic acid is a chemical peel that reduces the dead layers of skin. It is applied by a dermatologist but can also be found in some cosmetics.

Prescription topical antibiotics and antibacterials stop or slow the growth of bacteria that are plugging the area. Some are also anti-inflammatory.

Topical retinoids reduce the abnormal skin growth. They can stop the development of new whiteheads and blackheads by unplugging the existing ones and allowing other medications to enter and work.

Prescription oral antibiotics reduce the production of P. acnes and reduce inflammation.

Systemic retinoids (Isotretinoin-Accutane and a newly developed generic version) reduce the size of the oil glands so less sebum is produced. It also slows the growth of P. acnes.

Hormonal therapies that contain estrogen reduce sebum production by blocking the effect of the male hormone, testosterone.

THE MOST COMMON POSSIBLE SIDE EFFECTS

Over-the-Counter Medications

- Mild redness
- Stinging
- Peeling

Prescription Topical Medications

- Dryness of skin
- Peeling
- Burning
- Redness
- Itching
- Skin discoloration at the site of application

Prescription Oral Antibiotics

- Nausea
- Vomiting

- Stomach cramps
- Diarrhea
- Dizziness
- Increased skin sensitivity to sunlight

Systemic Retinoids

- Dry mouth or nose
- Nosebleeds
- Inflamed lips
- Eye problems
- Difficulty wearing contact lenses
- Crusting of skin
- Rash
- Itching
- Peeling skin on hands and feet
- Increased sensitivity to sunlight
- Hair thinning
- Upset stomach
- Tiredness
- Headache
- Bone or joint pain
- Potential for psychiatric problems

Hormonal Therapies

- Breast enlargement or tenderness
- Sexuality changes
- Bloating
- Stomach cramps
- Appetite changes
- Weight changes
- Uterine bleeding or spotting
- Nausea
- Unusual tiredness or weakness

- Diarrhea
- Reduced sperm count

OTHER PRECAUTIONS

Over-the-Counter Medications and Prescription Topical Medications

- Some topical acne medications contain alcohol that leads to the burning and stinging sensation on your skin. Do not use this medication near an open flame or while smoking. They might also stain your skin while you are using them, but it should go away when you stop.

- Benzoyl peroxide is a bleach that can affect your hair or clothing, so you need to be careful when using it to keep it away from your hair or your clothes.

- Many of these medications make you more susceptible to sunburn and this can cause additional problems over time such as premature aging of your skin or skin cancer. Stay away from the sun as much as possible and stay away from tanning booths and sun lamps.

Prescription Oral Antibiotics

- Some prescription oral antibiotics may reduce the effectiveness of oral contraceptives. You will need to use an additional form of birth control if you are taking these medications.

- Antacids can reduce the effectiveness of some oral antibiotics since the antibiotics combine with the antacids to form a substance that is too large to be able to pass through the walls of the intestine and enter the bloodstream.

- Some of these medications have been known to affect pregnancies and can pass into breast milk. Check with your doctor if you are pregnant or nursing.

Systemic Retinoids

- This medication has been known to cause serious birth defects. You *must not* become pregnant while taking this medication.

17

You must use two methods of birth control if you are sexually active and are taking this drug.

◎ This type of medication is only prescribed for the most severe form of acne (nodular acne) and only if all other treatments have been tried unsuccessfully. It is considered a last resort for severe acne.

◎ There have been reports of serious mental problems, including suicide, in people who are taking or who have taken this medication. Make sure you understand all risks.

◎ If you wear contact lenses, you may have difficulty since this medication can cause your eyes to be drier.

◎ Your skin might be more sensitive to the sun. Take precautions against sunlight and tanning booths.

Hormonal Therapies

◎ These medications may increase the risk of certain cancers.

◎ Cigarette smoking may increase the risk of certain side effects of these medications.

◎ These medications have been known to affect pregnancies and can pass into breast milk. Check with your doctor if you are pregnant or nursing.

THE BOTTOM LINE

There is no cure for acne and it will usually clear up by itself as you get older. You can try the over-the-counter remedies first. If you don't get the results you want, check with your pediatrician or a dermatologist. Make sure you discuss any other preparations you are using and follow the directions of those preparations carefully. All medications take time to work so you won't see results overnight. If you experience any of the side effects listed, or other problems that aren't listed, check with your doctor right away. There may be another remedy that will work better without the side effects you are experiencing. Even if your friend looks like he or she has the same type of acne, don't take a medication that was prescribed for someone else. Ask your doctor about it and see if it might be right for you.

Many of the medications can take up to two to three months to show results. Don't quit too early on anything that is prescribed for you. Give it time to see if it will work. Also, don't stop the medication if it seems that the acne has cleared up before you have completed the recommended dosage. This can cause the problem to return or get worse.

Some cosmetics and toiletry items can worsen the effects of acne medications. Try to use products labeled "noncomedogenic" that have been formulated so they will not cause acne. Cosmetics should be oil free.

Avoid foods that seem to worsen your acne. Although no specific food has been found to cause acne, you might find that yours gets worse if you eat chocolate or fried foods, for example. Keep a watch on this to see if it makes a difference for you.

There are new over-the-counter acne medications being developed regularly. They usually contain combinations of the products listed above. Check what they say they can do and check the ingredients used to see how they work.

Many of the topical applications come in cream, gel, or lotion. Check with your doctor about the right one for your type of skin.

Some medications that you take for other disorders can cause acne. If that happens, don't stop the medication. Talk with your doctor about what you can do to control the symptoms or see if there is another medication you can take that will not have this side effect.

Laser techniques are being developed to treat acne and the FDA has approved their use for acne on the back and face. According to the literature, they work by penetrating into your skin and creating a mild injury that changes the way your glands function. They report that results last for up to six months and the treatment may need to be repeated. The side effects are listed as minimal and include redness that does not last more than a few hours and slight changes in skin tone that could last a few weeks. There is also the possibility of pain associated with the treatments.

I take minocycline, an antibiotic, one or two per day. When I first started taking it, I thought it was a miracle. The acne disappeared. But my body got used to it and the acne started to come back. I take it when the acne builds up and the pimples go away after a couple of days. I feel like I have to take more and more to get it to work. If I have a big outbreak, I take more and it helps a lot. I try to take just enough to keep it manageable, so that I don't scream when I see myself in the mirror in the morning. I'm sporadic about taking medications. I take the antibiotic for a while and the acne will go away. Then I stop taking it and it comes back. I haven't told my doctor that I am doing it that way. I find that the beach or the desert when I visit my grandmother in Phoenix helps more than the medication.— Jeff, Atlanta, age 18

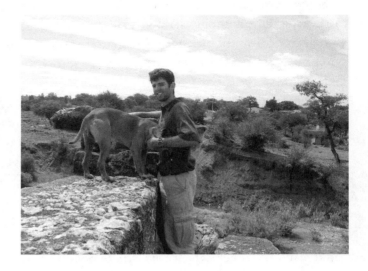

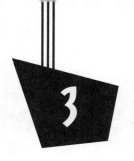

Attention Deficit Hyperactivity Disorder (ADHD)

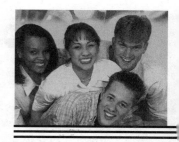

According to the National Institute of Mental Health, ADHD is a condition characterized by the behaviors of inattention, hyperactivity, and impulsivity over a period of time. It affects your ability to maintain focus and attention to a task. The behaviors are excessive and long term and occur in almost all situations.

THE MOST COMMON PRESCRIPTION MEDICATIONS

Stimulants

Methylphenidate—Short acting (Ritalin®)

Methylphenidate—Extended release (Concerta®)

Dextro-Amphetamine (Dexedrine®)

Pemoline (Cylert®)

Dextro-Amphetamine and Amphetamine (Adderall®)

Dexmethylphenidate (Focalin®)

Nonstimulant

Atomoxetine (Strattera®)

Tricyclic Antidepressants (TCAs)

Imipramine (Tofranil®)

Desipramine (Norpramin®)

Nortriptyline (Pamelor®)

MYTHS ABOUT STIMULANT MEDICATION

Myth:
Stimulants can lead to drug addiction later in life.
Fact:
Stimulants help many children focus and be more successful at school, home, and play. Avoiding negative experiences now may actually help prevent addictions and other emotional problems later.

Myth:
Responding well to a stimulant drug proves a person has ADHD.
Fact:
Stimulants allow many people to focus and pay better attention, whether or not they have ADHD. The improvement is just more noticeable in people with ADHD.

Myth:
Medication should be stopped when the child reaches adolescence.
Fact:
Not so! About 80 percent of those who needed medication as children still need it as teenagers. Fifty percent need medication as adults.

Reproduced by permission from the National Institute of Mental Health, www.nimh.nih.gov/publicat/adhd.cfm#adhd10, NIH Publication No. 96-3572, 1996.

GENERAL INFORMATION ABOUT HOW THESE DRUGS WORK

It is believed that ADHD is a result of an imbalance in the way your brain's neurotransmitters (brain chemicals that nerves use to communicate with each other) function. The medications that treat the symptoms of ADHD affect the way that the brain chemicals dopamine and norepinephrine are transmitted and used to help your nerves communicate with each other. The medications increase your ability to pay attention and decrease your tendency for impulsivity and hyperactivity. Most do not permanently change you or your brain and many of them are only effective for the amount of time indicated by the dose and type you take. The medications do not cure ADHD and they do not control your behavior. They enable you to function more effectively and changes are often your own strengths and abilities that are able to emerge.

I started taking Strattera® in the fall 2003. I take one tablet every morning. I tried other medications but they were not the right medications for me. I took Wellbutrin® from age eight to age twelve, but I gained a tolerance to it. The Strattera® helps a lot and my mood and energy levels are back to normal. I have a better memory and am better able to focus. When I am not on medication I am a lot more spontaneous and I procrastinate a lot. It is much more difficult to focus. One summer I did not take my medication. That summer a lot of bad things happened because I was spontaneous and I didn't think of what I was doing. My best friend and I were getting into trouble and because of that I lost my best friend. I am not allowed to see him any more. Now that I'm on medication, those things I did that summer, I never would have done if I had been on meds and the bad things never would have happened. I feel it is not wise if you know something will help and you choose not to let it.—Wesley, age 16, tenth grade

Stimulants are thought to affect the transmission of the neurotransmitter dopamine by stimulating the release of it. This activates the nerve cells and has the effect of decreasing restlessness and increasing attention and concentration.

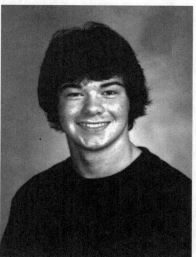

Atomoxetine is thought to affect the transmission of the neurotransmitter norepinephrine. It is believed to reduce the reabsorption of norepinephrine by the nerves and leaves more of it available to communicate with other nerves.

Tricyclic antidepressants affect the transmission of the neurotransmitters norepinephrine and dopamine. They block the passage of these chemicals as they go in and out of the nerve endings and raise the levels of them in the brain. This produces a sedative effect. It is possible that these medications change the way your nerve endings function over time.

This shows the connection between two neurons (the "synapse"). Dopamine is stored within the nerve endings of a neuron. Electrical impulses traveling down the axon toward the ending cause the release of dopamine into the synaptic space between the ending and the neighboring neuron. Once in the synaptic space, the dopamine binds to special proteins, called receptors, on the membrane of a neighboring neuron. When dopamine binds to dopamine receptors it causes a change in the electrical properties of the receiving neuron and the process of releasing the dopamine starts all over again. This is how neurons communicate with each other.

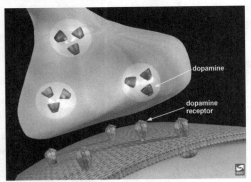

National Institute on Drug Abuse, *The Brain & the Actions of Cocaine, Opiates, and Marijuana—Slide Teaching Packet for Scientists* (Washington, DC: U.S. Department of Health and Human Services, National Institutes of Health, 2003).

THE MOST COMMON POSSIBLE SIDE EFFECTS

Stimulants

- Nervousness
- Trouble sleeping
- Loss of appetite
- Stomach pain
- Weight loss
- Irregular heartbeat
- Restlessness
- Dizziness

Nonstimulant

- Indigestion
- Nausea
- Vomiting
- Fatigue
- Decreased appetite
- Mood swings

Tricyclic Antidepressants

- Blurred vision
- Dry mouth
- Dizziness or lightheadedness
- Constipation
- Difficulty urinating
- Sensitivity to bright light
- Weight changes
- Drowsiness
- Headache
- Increased appetite
- Nausea
- Unpleasant taste

OTHER PRECAUTIONS

Stimulants

◎ Stimulants have the potential for being abused if they are not used correctly. Never let your friends take your medication and do not take something that was prescribed for someone else. Most of these medications have been studied for a long time and are considered safe if taken as directed and for the disorder prescribed.

◎ If you are taking a long-acting form of the medication, you may still need to take a short-acting form to cover crucial times that not covered by the longer acting one.

◎ Long-acting medications should never be crushed or chewed but swallowed whole.

◎ Stimulants may interact with psychotropic drugs, antihistamines, anticonvulsants, or other stimulants (e.g., caffeine) that excite your central nervous system and increase or decrease effectiveness of prescription stimulants or the other medications and/or cause additional side effects.

◎ These medications have been known to affect pregnancies and can pass into breast milk. Check with your doctor if you are pregnant or nursing.

I took Ritalin® from first grade until sixth grade. It made me feel bad and my parents described me as being angry. Concerta® feels like having a cup of coffee. It helps me concentrate. The hardest part is paying attention in math class. If you have something extra to help you improve note taking and grades, it's a worthwhile investment. I take a small dose and don't notice side effects. If a drug doesn't feel right, I stop taking it. I only take it during the week for school. It is a great way to get through the school day. Everything takes longer when I am not on Concerta®, but it is nice to take longer on the weekends.—Jeffrey, age 18

- ◎ These medications can make you drowsy. Make sure you know how they affect you before you do anything that requires your full alertness.
- ◎ These medications have been known to cause an increase in tics associated with Tourette Syndrome.
- ◎ Pemoline has been known to cause liver damage. If this is the medication that works for you, be sure your liver function is carefully monitored by your prescribing doctor.

Nonstimulant

- ◎ There have been incidences of impaired sexual function in some people taking this medication.

Tricyclic Antidepressants

- ◎ Smoking and oral contraceptives may reduce the effects of TCAs.
- ◎ These medications can add to the effects of alcohol and other central nervous system depressants.
- ◎ These medications have been known to affect pregnancies and can pass into breast milk. Check with your doctor if you are pregnant or nursing.
- ◎ These medications can make your skin more sensitive to the sun. Make sure you take proper precautions when in the sun and avoid tanning booths and sun lamps.

THE BOTTOM LINE

There are other conditions that appear to have the same symptoms as ADHD. Make sure you have an accurate diagnosis before beginning medication for ADHD. Just because your friend has the same symptoms and got the diagnosis of ADHD, it doesn't mean that you have it.

Stimulants are usually the first medication tried for ADHD. Methylphenidate was approved in 1955 and it has been studied extensively. If stimulants do not work, or if you have severe side effects, one of the other medications listed may be tried. Also,

> I have taken Adderall® since sixth grade. Before I took it, I was considered a disruptive child. I talked a lot and wandered off in my own little world. When I started taking it, I felt weird having to take medication for a condition. Then I noticed I was doing better in school so I was okay with it. I was surprised when report cards came out, but realized why—that I was able to pay attention in class. I can definitely concentrate easier. Social studies is not the most exciting class and it is easier to pay attention in that class. I take it during the week and on weekends. I also take it over vacations because the side effects are worse if I don't take it all the time. It definitely helps. Just taking a little pill once a day—it does a lot.— Robert, age 14

your doctor may try a combination of medications to find what works for you.

Other disorders that are associated with ADHD are learning disabilities, Tourette Syndrome, oppositional defiant disorder, conduct disorder, anxiety, or depression, and the medications taken for ADHD should be tailored to take other conditions into account.

If your school requires that the school nurse give all medications, you may be called to the nurse's office during the day to take your pill. You may be able to avoid that if you can take one of the longer acting types so that it will last through the whole school day.

ADHD is rarely treated with medication alone, but medication is a major part of the treatment. The treatment needs to be combined with the appropriate educational program and you might also benefit from psychological counseling to talk about the effects ADHD has had on your life. You need to remain actively involved with your doctors, your teachers, and your parents to monitor your educational and medication needs. A medication diary (see the Medication Diary form at the end of the book) may be useful to help determine if there are interfering side effects.

> I didn't ask about the medication. I knew what it was supposed to do. It helped me concentrate more and helped me focus and keep my attention longer in the day. The doctor told me about the side effects but they weren't true for me. Most of my friends are on it, so it wasn't a problem. The biggest difference is when I read. I hate reading. I can read for two hours without getting antsy. No one knows you are taking it if you don't tell them. I am going away to college next year and I had to tell the school. I don't know if they will let me take it on my own or if I will have to go to the school nurse each day. That would be a pain.—Adam, age 18, takes Concerta® once a day

You should have regular checkups with your doctor while you are on any of these medications.

ADHD doesn't just affect your life in school. If you are involved in after-school activities that require attention or social demands, you may want to be sure that your medication is working while you take part in the fun things, too.

Some of your friends may not take their medication on weekends when they do not need to concentrate like you do in

> I have been taking Concerta® for about two years. I took others, but one of those made me go to sleep. With Concerta® you can concentrate on one subject—like schoolwork. I am not as social. It helped me a lot in school. I don't take it on weekends and I am not as concentrated then. I didn't want to take it at first, but once you get to high school and your grades go down, you realize it is worth taking because it boosts your grades. My advice to others is TAKE IT! It is no big deal in high school.— Jim, age 15, ninth grade

school. That is a something you need to discuss with your doctor and the decision is based on you and your lifestyle. If you play team sports on the weekend, you may need to be on the medication in order to focus on your game. If you do long-term homework assignments on the weekend, you may need the medication to help you concentrate. On the other hand, the weekend may be a time to see how you do without the medication. Make your decision on well thought out considerations and don't be swayed by what your friends are doing.

Medication for ADHD is not a crutch. It is something you need in order to perform better in your life and is similar to a need for glasses or braces.

Cephalon, Inc., an international biopharmaceutical company, is studying the use of the narcolepsy drug Provigil® for the treatment of the symptoms of ADHD. The first study showed significant improvement in the symptoms with the following side effects: mild to moderate insomnia, abdominal pain, loss of appetite, cough, and fever. The most common complaint was headaches. The advantages are that it might help in cases where the stimulants are not effective and it does not appear to cause the same weight-loss problems as stimulants.

There are other medications prescribed for ADHD that are off-label uses, such as the atypical antidepressant Bupropion (Wellbutrin®) and the antihypertensives Clonidine (Catapres®) and Guanfacine (Tenex®). Off-label means that they are not currently approved for ADHD by the Food and Drug Administration (FDA); however, some physicians feel they show benefit for this condition.

Bupropion (Wellbutrin®) mildly slows down the action of certain neurotransmitters. For information about side effects and other precautions of this type of medication, see the chapter 7 on depression.

Antihypertensives stimulate nerve endings in the brain by affecting the neurotransmitter norepinephrine. A side effect of this type of medication is sedation and it is for this reason that it is used in the treatment of ADHD. It appears to treat the hyperactivity associated with ADHD and the sleep problems that are a side effect of stimulant medications. They are often given in combination with stimulants for maximum effect. For information about the side effects and other precautions of this type of medication, see chapter 18 on Tourette Syndrome.

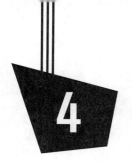

4 Allergies

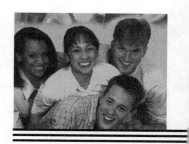

Allergies are harmful sensitivities to particular substances. They show up with exposure to substances in the air such as pollen, pet dander, or dust; exposure to certain foods such as peanuts or fish; exposure to things on your skin such as wool, latex, or poison ivy; insect stings; and exposure to certain medications like penicillin or sulfa. (Asthma and eczema are included in separate sections.)

THE MOST COMMON OVER-THE-COUNTER (OTC) AND PRESCRIPTION MEDICATIONS

Antihistamines

Over-the-Counter

Diphenhydramine (Benadryl®)

Chlorpheniramine (Chlor-Trimeton®)

Clemastine (Tavist®)

Loratadine (Claritin®)

Prescription

Fexofenadine (Allegra®)

Desloratadine (Clarinex®)

Azelastine (Astelin®)

Cetirizine (Zyrtec®)

Decongestants

Over-the-Counter

Pseudoephedrine (Sudafed®)

Phenylephrine (Neo-Synephrine Nasal Spray®)

Oxymetazoline (Afrin 12 Hour Nasal Spray®)

Prescription Nasal Spray

Tetrahydrozoline (Tyzine®)

Prescription Combinations of Antihistamine Plus Decongestant

Fexofenadine and Pseudoephedrine (Allegra D®)

Prescription Inhaled Mast Cell Stabilizers

Cromolyn Sodium (NasalCrom®)

Nedocromil (Alocril®)

Prescription Anti-Inflammatory Agents

Corticosteroids—Oral

Prednisone (Deltasone®)

Corticosteroids—Nasal Sprays

Fluticasone (Flonase®)

Triamcinolone (Nasacort®)

Budesonide (Rhinocort®)

Flunisolide (Nasalide®)

Beclomethasone (Beconase®)

Mometasone (Nasonex®)

Prescription Leukotriene Modifiers

Montelukast (Singulair®)

Zafirlukast (Accolate®)

Zileuton (Zyflo®)

Prescription Sympathomimetic Agents

Epinephrine (Epipen®)

Eye Drops

Prescription Antihistamine/Mass Cell Stabilizer

Olopatadine (Patanol®)

Levocabastine (Livostin®)

Emedastine (Emadine®)

Azelastine (Optivar®)

Lodoxamide (Alomide®)

OTC Combinations of Antihistamine Plus Decongestant

Naphazoline and Pheniramine (Visine-A®)

OTC Nonsteroidal Anti-Inflammatory Drugs (NSAID)

Ketorolac (Acular®)

GENERAL INFORMATION ABOUT HOW THESE DRUGS WORK

When an irritant (allergen) stimulates your immune system, your white blood cells produce antibodies to attack the irritant. In some cases, this action may also release histamines, prostaglandins, and leukotrienes (chemicals that occur naturally in the body and can bind to other cells causing inflammation) that cause the symptoms of an allergic reaction. There is no cure for allergies, but medications can reduce allergic symptoms.

Antihistamines block the action of histamines that are released when your body encounters an allergen. They dry up secretions in your nose, throat, and eyes. This helps relieve or prevent the sneezing, itchy eyes and throat, and postnasal drip that the histamine may cause.

Decongestants narrow the blood vessels and reduce the blood flow into the swollen tissues of your nose. This reduces the secretions from your nose, shrinks the swollen tissues, and improves your airflow.

Mast cell stabilizers—inhaled and eye drops—prevent the release of histamines and other chemicals from the mast cells by stabilizing the mast cells. Mast cells are a key cause of allergic reactions because they are the cells that release the chemicals that cause the symptoms.

Corticosteroids and anti-inflammatory eye drops block the release of chemicals in the body that produce inflammation. The corticosteroids also block some of your immune system's response to irritants.

Corticosteroid nasal sprays work on the lining of the airways. They block the cause of the inflammation there and reduce the immune system's response to the irritants that are inhaled. They also block the secretion of mucus in the airways.

Leukotriene modifiers are anti-inflammatories that block leukotriene from forming or, if formed, from binding to the receptor cells so that inflammation can't occur.

Epinephrine, which is given by injection in the case of anaphylactic shock, is a sympathomimetic agent that opens the airways to the lungs and improves blood circulation by relaxing the muscles that surround the airways. It mimics your body's automatic response to fight stress or an emergency situation.

Antihistamine and decongestant eye drops relieve the redness, itchiness, and watery eyes associated with allergy symptoms.

THE MOST COMMON POSSIBLE SIDE EFFECTS

OTC Antihistamines

- Drowsiness
- Stomach distress
- Dry mouth
- Thickening of mucus

Prescription Antihistamines

- ◎ Drowsiness
- ◎ Dry mouth
- ◎ Bitter taste in the mouth
- ◎ Headache
- ◎ Nausea

OTC Decongestants

- ◎ Nervousness
- ◎ Restlessness
- ◎ Sleeplessness

Prescription Decongestant Nasal Sprays

- ◎ Burning, dryness, or stinging inside the nose
- ◎ Severe nasal obstruction with repeated use

Combinations of Antihistamine Plus Decongestant

- ◎ Restlessness
- ◎ Nervousness
- ◎ Sleeplessness
- ◎ Excitability
- ◎ Dizziness
- ◎ Headache

Inhaled Mast Cell Stabilizers

- ◎ Throat irritation
- ◎ Cough

Corticosteroids—Oral

- ◎ Short Term:
  - ◎ Fluid retention and weight gain
  - ◎ Slow healing of wounds

◎ Easy bruising

◎ Increased appetite

◎ Indigestion

◎ Long Term:

  ◎ Slow growth

  ◎ Lowered resistance to infections

  ◎ Eye problems (including cataracts)

  ◎ Headache

  ◎ Muscle weakness

  ◎ Unusual increase in facial hair growth

  ◎ Menstruation problems

  ◎ Thinning skin

Corticosteroids—Nasal Sprays

◎ Irritation of throat

◎ Burning and dryness or other irritation inside nose

Leukotriene Modifiers

◎ Headache

Sympathomimetic Agents

◎ Headache

◎ Tremors

Eye Drops

◎ Stinging or burning when applied

◎ Headache

OTHER PRECAUTIONS

Antihistamines

◎ These medications can add to the effects of alcohol and other central nervous system depressants.

◎ Even if you are taking over-the-counter medication, you should do it in conjunction with your doctor's advice to make sure you get the proper dosage and to make sure the medication will not interact adversely with any other medication or condition you have.

OTC Decongestants

◎ These medications have been known to affect pregnancies and can pass into breast milk. Check with your doctor if you are pregnant or nursing.

Prescription Decongestant Nasal Sprays

◎ Nasal sprays or nose drops should be used for acute situations only. They should not be used for more than two or three days in a row or they may cause an increase in the symptoms they are trying to treat.

Combinations of Antihistamine Plus Decongestant

◎ These medications may pass into breast milk. You may want to consider bottle-feeding if you are taking this type of medication.

Corticosteroids—Oral

◎ Corticosteroids should not be stopped without supervision from your doctor. Abruptly stopping this type of medication can have serious side effects.

◎ Because long-term use of corticosteroids lowers your resistance to infections, check with your doctor before having a vaccination or before making plans to be with others who have been vaccinated.

◎ Oral contraceptives may also increase the side effects of corticosteroids.

◎ These medications have been known to affect pregnancies and can pass into breast milk. Check with your doctor if you are pregnant or nursing.

Corticosteroids—Nasal Sprays

◎ These medications may pass into breast milk. You may want to consider bottle-feeding if you are taking this type of medication.

Leukotriene Modifiers

◎ These medications have been known to affect pregnancies and can pass into breast milk. Check with your doctor if you are pregnant or nursing.

◎ These medications may help reduce the number of attacks you have. They do not help once an attack has occurred.

◎ Alcohol use can increase serious side effects of this type of medication.

Sympathomimetic Agents

◎ These medications have been known to affect pregnancies and can pass into breast milk. Check with your doctor if you are pregnant or nursing.

◎ If your allergy is life threatening, wear a medical alert bracelet or necklace to identify your allergy and what to do in an emergency. You should always carry an epinephrine injection kit if that is what you need in an emergency.

◎ After taking the epinephrine shot, you should go to a hospital or emergency facility immediately. There is always the danger of a second wave of the symptoms following your initial attack.

Eye Drops

◎ If you wear contact lenses, you should wait at least fifteen minutes after using eye drops before inserting your contacts. Talk with your doctor and optometrist about other precautions regarding contact lenses. Some of the medications should not be used at all with contact lenses.

◎ These medications have been known to affect pregnancies and can pass into breast milk. Check with your doctor if you are pregnant or nursing.

THE BOTTOM LINE

The first step for controlling allergies is to try to stay away from what is causing them. If that is not possible, check with your doctor about allergy medications that might be right for you. Your allergy may be different from your friends, so the allergy medication your friend uses might not be the right medication or the right dosage for you.

Some of the medications must be taken on a regular basis to reduce the number of allergy attacks you have and some of them work once the attack has occurred. You may need to take more than one type of medication depending upon the type of allergic reaction you have.

Immunotherapy can modify the way your immune system reacts to the allergy-causing irritants. It is used when the source of your allergy can be positively identified and/or it is not possible for you to avoid that source and other remedies have not been successful. This is done through shots given by your doctor. It helps you build immunity to the source of the allergy by increasing your body's ability to produce a protective antibody to fight the antibody that causes the allergy symptoms. Side effects of the shots may include swelling and irritations at the site of the injection as well as itchy eyes, shortness of breath, runny nose, and a tight throat.

Scientists are currently developing shots designed to interact with IgE (immunoglobulin E), a type of antibody produced by immune system cells that can causes allergic reactions. The medication would block the IgE antibody from triggering the allergic reaction. One of these medications, Omalizumab, is approved for asthma but not yet for other allergies. Another is TNX-901 that is awaiting approval for peanut allergies. The initial trials show them to be safe and well tolerated.

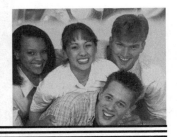

Anxiety Disorders

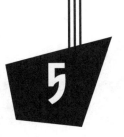

5

Anxiety disorders are a group of conditions that are closely related. The general characteristics are excessive, irrational, and pervasive fear or dread about a variety of objects or situations that causes a disruption in your ability to function in your daily life. The major types of anxiety disorders are Panic Disorder, Obsessive-Compulsive Disorder, Post-Traumatic Stress Disorder, Phobias, Generalized Anxiety Disorder, and Social Anxiety Disorder.

THE MOST COMMON PRESCRIPTION MEDICATIONS

Antianxiety Medications

Benzodiazepines

Clonazepam (Klonopin®)

Alprazolam (Xanax®)

Diazepam (Valium®)

Lorazepam (Ativan®)

Azaspirones

Buspirone (BuSpar®)

Antidepressants

Selective Serotonin Reuptake Inhibitors (SSRIs)

Fluoxetine (Prozac®)

Fluvoxamine (Luvox®)

Paroxetine (Paxil®)

Sertraline (Zoloft®)

Citalopram (Celexa®)

Atypical Antidepressants

Venlafaxine (Effexor®)

Trazodone (Desyrel®)

Nefazodone (Serzone®)

Monoamine Oxidase Inhibitors (MAOIs)

Phenelzine (Nardil®)

Tranylcypromine (Parnate®)

Tricyclic Antidepressants (TCAs)

Imipramine (Tofranil®)

Amitriptyline (Elavil®)

Nortriptyline (Pamelor®)

Desipramine (Norpramin®)

Clomipramine (Anafranil®)

Beta-Blockers

Propranolol (Inderal®)

Mood Stabilizers

Gabapentin (Neurontin®)

Valproic Acid (Depakene®)

Ancient Greeks created cures for anxiety by interpreting dreams. The early Chinese used finger pressure on trigger points in the hands. Dian Dincin Buchman, *Ancient Healing Secrets: Practical Cures That Work Today* (Baltimore: Ottenheimer, 1996).

GENERAL INFORMATION ABOUT HOW THESE DRUGS WORK

Anxiety disorders are believed to occur due to a combination of genetic and environmental factors. Different parts of the brain

41

and different chemicals in the brain appear to have an influence. The amygdala, a small structure deep inside the brain that coordinates your body's fear response, is involved in some types of anxiety disorders. The neurotransmitter, serotonin, and the brain chemicals gamma-aminobutyric acid (GABA) and Substance P also appear to be linked to anxiety disorders. Certain hormone imbalances are also implicated. Medications are used (along with therapeutic counseling) to treat the symptoms of the disorder by targeting the specific neurotransmitters, brain chemical, or hormones.

Benzodiazepines are central nervous system depressants. They slow down your nervous system by helping GABA inhibit activity in some of the nerves in the brain.

The way that Azaspirones (Buspirone®) works is not fully known. It is thought to decrease the action of serotonin in the brain. It does not have the same potential for addictions as other antianxiety medications.

SSRIs keep the neurotransmitter serotonin from being absorbed by your cells and keeps it in the spaces surrounding the nerve endings of the cells in your brain. That way the action of the serotonin is increased and that helps improve your mood.

The exact way the atypical antidepressants (those that don't fit well into any other medication category) work is not fully understood at this time. They are thought to balance the levels of certain neurotransmitters, such as serotonin, norepinephrine, and dopamine, which are linked to mood, emotion, and mental state.

MAOIs block the action of monoamine oxidase, an enzyme in your body that breaks down certain hormones. This allows the amount of the hormones to increase and provides a therapeutic effect.

TCAs affect the levels of the neurotransmitters norepinephrine and serotonin. These neurotransmitters are linked to mood, emotion, and mental state. The antidepressants block the passage of these chemicals as they go in and out of the nerve endings and this produces a sedative effect and can elevate mood. It is possible that these medications change the way your nerve endings function over time.

Beta-blockers interfere with the action of the part of the nervous system that controls the pace of your heart. They reduce your heart rate and lower your blood pressure.

The way the mood stabilizers work is also not fully understood. It is thought that they interfere with the reuptake (absorption) of certain neurotransmitters and affect the way the nerves communicate with each other. They allow more of the neurotransmitters to remain in your brain so that they are more available to reduce depressive and manic episodes. The increased amount of neurotransmitters available can also have a stabilizing effect on your mood.

THE MOST COMMON POSSIBLE SIDE EFFECTS

Benzodiazepines

- Drowsiness
- Unsteadiness
- Dizziness
- Lightheadedness
- Slurred speech

Azaspirones

- Dizziness
- Nausea
- Headache
- Nervousness
- Lightheadedness
- Unusual excitement

This shows the anatomy of a neuron, the nerve cells that make up the pathways of your brain. The dendrites and soma (the body of the cell) receive chemical information from neighboring neuronal axons. The chemical information is converted to electrical currents that travel toward and converge on the soma. A major impulse is produced and travels down the axon toward the terminal. This is how the parts of the brain send and integrate information.

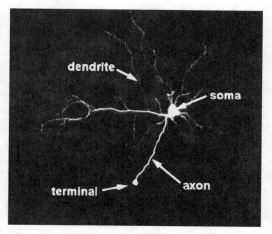

National Institute on Drug Abuse, *The Brain & the Actions of Cocaine, Opiates, and Marijuana—Slide Teaching Packet for Scientists* (Washington, DC: U.S. Department of Health and Human Services, National Institutes of Health, 2003).

SSRIs

- Headache
- Anxiety
- Nervousness
- Sleeplessness
- Drowsiness
- Tiredness
- Weakness
- Changes in sex drive
- Tremors
- Sweating
- Appetite loss
- Nausea
- Diarrhea
- Skin rash
- Itching

Atypical Antidepressants

- Constipation
- Bad taste in the mouth
- Nausea
- Vomiting
- Blood pressure changes
- Dizziness
- Confusion
- Drowsiness
- Fatigue
- Lightheadedness
- Sleeplessness
- Agitation
- Blurred vision
- Sexual problems
- Dry mouth

- Headache
- Tremors
- Weakness
- Increased sweating
- Loss of appetite

MAOIs

- Dizziness or lightheadedness (especially standing from lying or sitting)
- Headache
- Tremors
- Muscle twitching
- Sleeplessness
- Weakness
- Restlessness
- Drowsiness
- Nausea
- Weight changes
- Sexual difficulties
- Appetite changes (including craving for sweets)

TCAs

- Blurred vision
- Dry mouth
- Dizziness or lightheadedness
- Constipation
- Difficulty urinating
- Sensitivity to bright light
- Weight changes
- Drowsiness
- Headache
- Increased appetite
- Nausea
- Unpleasant taste in the mouth

Beta-Blockers

- ◎ Sexual difficulties
- ◎ Dizziness or lightheadedness
- ◎ Drowsiness
- ◎ Sleeplessness
- ◎ Unusual tiredness or weakness

Mood Stabilizers

- ◎ Drowsiness
- ◎ Dizziness
- ◎ Unusual tiredness or weakness
- ◎ Abnormal eye movements or twitching
- ◎ Vision problems
- ◎ Skin rash
- ◎ Nausea
- ◎ Vomiting
- ◎ Indigestion
- ◎ Unusual weight changes
- ◎ Loss of appetite
- ◎ Tremors
- ◎ Diarrhea

Many medications are tested on animals before they are tested on humans. It is difficult to do that with anxiety medications because laboratory animals regard researchers as a danger and feel anxious every time they are picked up. In order to judge whether the animal is responding to antianxiety medications, researchers have to measure actions such as muscle relaxation, increased or slowed heartbeats and breathing and a reduction of their twitching response.

Adapted from Alfred Burger, *Drugs and People, Medications, Their History and Origins, and the Way They Act* (Charlottesville: University Press of Virginia, 1986).

- Hair loss
- Unsteadiness

OTHER PRECAUTIONS

Benzodiazepines

- Benzodiazepines are generally prescribed for short periods of time because you can develop a tolerance to them. That would mean that you would have to stop taking the medication or the dosage would have to be increased.
- They also can become habit forming if taken for a long period of time. Be alert to signs that this happening.
- These medications have been known to affect pregnancies and can pass into breast milk. Check with your doctor if you are pregnant or nursing.
- These medications can add to the effects of alcohol and other central nervous system depressants.

Azaspirones

- This type of medication may take longer to take effect.

SSRIs

- There has been a lot of controversy concerning prescribing these medications for patients under the age of eighteen. Work closely with your doctor if SSRIs have been prescribed for you.
- Do not stop taking antidepressants without talking with your doctor. Some of them have side effects that occur if you stop abruptly and you may need to taper off the medication.
- These medications have been known to affect pregnancies and can pass into breast milk. Check with your doctor if you are pregnant or nursing.
- These medications can add to the effects of alcohol and other central nervous system depressants.

Atypical Antidepressants

- These medications can make you drowsy. Make sure you know how they affect you before you do anything that requires your full alertness.

⊚ These medications can add to the effects of alcohol and other central nervous system depressants.

⊚ These medications have been known to affect pregnancies and can pass into breast milk. Check with your doctor if you are pregnant or nursing.

⊚ Do not take these medications at or near the same time as you take MAOIs.

⊚ Serzone®, an atypical antidepressant that is not included in this list, has been taken off the market in the United States and other countries because of the risk of liver failure. Make sure you monitor this if Serzone® is working for you.

MAOIS

⊚ MAOIs are rarely used in children because of the restrictions to what you can eat. When taking MAOIs you need to avoid certain foods like pickles, many cheeses and wine, and decongestant medication due to the risk of an increase in blood pressure from the interaction of the tyramine in the food and the MAO inhibitors. You may need to be on a special diet if you are taking MAOIs.

⊚ You should not take MAOIs and other types of medications, especially those that increase the activity of serotonin, together or within a certain time period.

⊚ These medications can add to the effects of alcohol and other central nervous system depressants and could cause serious side effects.

TCAS

⊚ Smoking and oral contraceptives may reduce the effects of TCAs.

⊚ These medications can add to the effects of alcohol and other central nervous system depressants.

⊚ These medications have been known to affect pregnancies and can pass into breast milk. Check with your doctor if you are pregnant or nursing.

⊚ These medications can make your skin more sensitive to the sun. Make sure you take proper precautions when in the sun and avoid tanning booths and sun lamps.

Beta-Blockers

- ◎ These medications can make you drowsy. Make sure you know how they affect you before you do anything that requires your full alertness.

- ◎ These medications have been known to affect pregnancies and can pass into breast milk. Check with your doctor if you are pregnant or nursing.

Mood Stabilizers

- ◎ These medications can add to the effects of alcohol and other central nervous system depressants.

- ◎ These medications have been known to affect pregnancies and can pass into breast milk. Check with your doctor if you are pregnant or nursing.

THE BOTTOM LINE

Anxiety disorders are usually treated with psychotherapy as well as medication. Make sure you find someone you are comfortable with who can help you through therapy as well as be able to prescribe the medication that is right for you.

Not all anxiety disorders respond to the same medications. Your doctor is the one who can tell which medication is the right one for you. Don't share medications with friends, even if it seems they have the same diagnosis.

Medication does not cure the anxiety disorder. It will help you keep the symptoms under control so that you can lead a normal life without the disruptions caused by the anxiety.

It is possible to have other disorders, such as an eating disorder or depression, as well as the anxiety disorder. Your doctor should be able to treat all disorders at the same time.

Many of these medications are used in combinations and many cannot be combined. Your doctor knows which work well together and which don't. What works for your friend may not be the right combination for you, so comparing symptoms and medications is not a good idea.

Make sure your teachers and the school nurse know about your anxiety disorder and the medications you are taking. You may need accommodations if there are requirements that you cannot fulfill due to the side effects of the medications. You might need to postpone machine shop or driver's education while you are on medications that affect your concentration.

There has been a lot of publicity about whether Paxil and other SSRIs cause suicide. At this point doctors don't know whether it is the result of the medications or is the result of the condition. However, it should make you more alert to questions about the medication you are using. A good working relationship with your doctor is especially important when you are on medications for anxiety disorders.

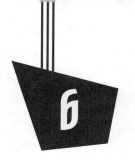

Asthma

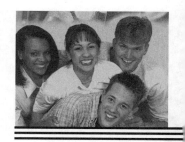

Asthma is a condition where bronchial tubes (airways to the lungs) are overly sensitive to certain environmental or internal factors and become narrower and mucus filled in response to irritants. These factors also cause the airways to become inflamed and it is difficult for air to enter and exit the lungs the way it should.

THE MOST COMMON PRESCRIPTION MEDICATIONS

Inhaled Bronchodilators

Short-Acting Beta-2 Agonists

Albuterol (Proventil®)
Pirbuterol (Maxair®)
Levalbuterol (Xopenex®)

Long-Acting Beta-2 Agonists

Salmeterol (Serevent®)
Formoterol (Foradil®)

Combinations

Salmeterol and Fluticasone (Advair Diskus®)
Albuterol Sulfate and Ipratroprium Bromide (Combivent®)

Anticholinergic

Ipratropium (Atrovent®)

Systemic Bronchodilators

Theophylline (Elixophyllin®)

Inhaled Anti-Inflammatory Medications

Corticosteroids

Beclomethasone (Vanceril®)

Fluticasone (Flovent®)

Budesonide (Pulmicort®)

Flunisolide (Aerobid®)

Triamcinolone (Azmacort®)

Mast Cell Stabilizers

Cromolyn (NasalCrom®)

Nedocromil (Alocril®)

Systemic Anti-Inflammatory Medications

Corticosteroids

Prednisolone (Prelone®)

Prednisone (Deltasone®)

Methylprednisolone (Medrol®)

Triamcinolone (Aristocort®)

Hydrocortisone (Hydrocortone®)

Leukotriene Modifiers

Zafirlukast (Accolate®)

Montelukast (Singulair®)

Zileuton (Zyflo®)

Monoclonal Antibody

Omalizumab (Xolair®)

GENERAL INFORMATION ABOUT HOW THESE DRUGS WORK

These medications are delivered in two different ways. They are either in pill form or inhaled. The inhaled forms are delivered through a nebulizer that delivers the medication in a mist, through a dry powder inhaler, or through a metered dose inhaler. They are either fast acting or for long-term control. The fast-acting forms work right away to control the immediate symptoms. The slower acting types do not provide relief of immediate symptoms, but work over time to control the frequency and severity of the symptoms. It is important to know which types of medications to take for your short- and long-term symptoms.

Most inhaled bronchodilators are fast acting and are for routine use, for severe asthma episodes, and for prevention of exercise-induced asthma. They work by opening the airways to the lungs by relaxing the surrounding muscles. The long-acting forms also block the release of histamines that narrow the airways but these do not work right way and are not to be used for an acute asthma attack. They are used on a regular basis for prevention.

> **Early Romans used raw garlic and garlic juice to treat asthma.** Dian Dincin Buchman, *Ancient Healing Secrets* (New York: Random House, 1996).

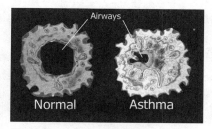

Airways before and after an Asthma Episode
Michelle Meadows, "Breathing Better: Action Plans Keep Asthma in Check." U.S. Food and Drug Administration, *FDA Consumer Magazine*, March–April 2003.

Advair Diskus® and Combivent® are bronchodilators with two types of inhaled chemicals joined to have a combined effect. Advair Diskus® combines a long-acting Beta-2 agonist with a corticosteroid. It works to open the airways and reduce inflammation. Combivent® is a short-acting Beta-2 agonist and an anticholinergic. It works to open the airways and to decrease coughing and wheezing.

Anticholinergics block the action of acetylcholine. This is a chemical that, in the lungs, causes the muscles around the airways to constrict. When the action is blocked, the airways widen or dilate. This decreases coughing and wheezing.

Systemic bronchodilator medications are used for severe episodes and chronic severe asthma that can't be controlled by the other types of medications. They control asthma by relaxing the bronchial (airways) muscles to open the airways and increasing the flow of air.

Anti-inflammatory medications are usually given daily to stop inflammation of the airways. They are the cornerstones of treatment. Even though you do not feel the airways opening and the immediate relief that is felt with beta agonists, long-term use of anti-inflammatories will make you have fewer episodes of asthma attacks. (Always have your short-acting inhalant medication at hand for immediate relief of an attack.) Once the inflammation is controlled, the obstruction and sensitivity in the airways is reduced. The inhalers can prevent attacks if used regularly, but they cannot relieve the attack once it starts. The inhalers work by preventing the cells in the lungs from releasing substances that cause the asthma symptoms. The dosage of an inhaler can be less than a systemic anti-inflammatory because the drug goes directly to the lungs. Also, there are fewer side effects with the inhaler than with the systemic type.

Mast cell stabilizers prevent the mast cells from releasing chemicals that can cause swelling and inflammation. They must be used on a regular basis to be effective or just before exposure.

Corticosteroids block the release of chemicals in the body that produce inflammation and suppress the activity of your immune system.

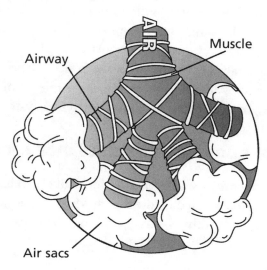

Before an Asthma Episode

Airway

Muscle

Air sacs

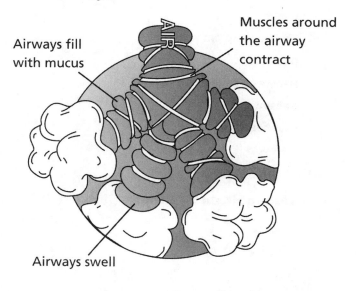

After an Asthma Episode

Airways fill
with mucus

Muscles around
the airway
contract

Airways swell

Infographic: FDA/Renée Gordon

Normal and Asthma-Affected Airways
With permission from National Institute of Allergy and Infectious Diseases,
National Institutes of Health (NIH) Asthma Basics, www.niaid.nih.gov/
newsroom/focuson/asthma01/basics.htm, August 30, 2001.

Leukotriene modifiers are anti-inflammatories that block leukotriene (chemicals that occur naturally in the body and can bind to other cells causing inflammation) from forming or, if formed, from binding to the receptor cells so that inflammation can't occur.

Omalizumab is taken by injection. It neutralizes an antibody in the immune system that can trigger the release of histamine. It can prevent attacks rather than controlling systems.

THE MOST COMMON POSSIBLE SIDE EFFECTS

Oral, or systemic, medications are more likely to have side effects than the inhaled medications. Most of the side effects listed are usually only evident with long-term use.

Inhaled Bronchodilators

- Nervousness
- Dry mouth or throat
- Cough
- Flu-like symptoms
- Dizziness
- Headache
- Nausea
- Fast heartbeat
- Tremors

Systemic Bronchodilators

- Nausea
- Vomiting
- Diarrhea
- Irritability
- Sleeplessness
- Fast heartbeat

Inhaled Anti-Inflammatory Corticosteroid Medications

- Dry mouth
- Hoarseness
- Cough
- Thrush is common if mouth is not rinsed after use

Inhaled Mast Cell Stabilizers

- Throat irritation
- Cough

Oral Corticosteroids

- Short term:
    - Fluid retention and weight gain
    - Slow healing of wounds
    - Easy bruising
    - Increased appetite
    - Indigestion
    - Insomnia
- Long term:
    - Slow growth
    - Lowered resistance to infections
    - Eye problems (including cataracts)
    - Headache
    - Muscle weakness
    - Unusual increase in facial hair growth
    - Menstruation problems
    - Thinning skin

Leukotriene Modifiers

- Headache

Monoclonal Antibody

- Injection-site reaction
- Cold symptoms
- Headache
- Joint pain
- Fatigue

OTHER PRECAUTIONS

Inhaled Bronchodilators

- It is easy to overuse inhaled reliever medications and that can worsen your condition. Take these medications only as prescribed by your doctor. If the prescribed dose is not effective, call your doctor. Do not take more!
- These medications have been known to affect pregnancies and can pass into breast milk. Check with your doctor if you are pregnant or nursing.

Systemic Bronchodilators

- Caffeine may increase the side effects of systemic and inhaled bronchodilators.
- These medications have been known to affect pregnancies and can pass into breast milk. Check with your doctor if you are pregnant or nursing.

Inhaled Mast Cell Stabilizers

- These medications need to be taken at the same time every day in order to have maximum effectiveness. They also need to be taken even if your asthma appears to be better. Plan your dose times when it will be convenient on a regular basis.

Oral Corticosteroids

- Corticosteroids should not be stopped without supervision from your doctor. Abruptly stopping this type of medication can have serious side effects.

- Because long-term use of corticosteroids lowers your resistance to infections, check with your doctor before having a vaccination or before making plans to be with others who have been vaccinated.
- Oral contraceptives may also increase the side effects of corticosteroids.
- These medications have been known to affect pregnancies and can pass into breast milk. Check with your doctor if you are pregnant or nursing.

Leukotriene Modifiers

- These medications have been known to affect pregnancies and can pass into breast milk. Check with your doctor if you are pregnant or nursing.
- These medications may help reduce the number of attacks you have. They do not help once an attack has occurred.
- Alcohol use can increase serious side effects of this type of medication.

Monoclonal Antibody

- There is not a lot of information known about how this medication affects pregnancy and nursing. Check this out with your doctor if you are pregnant or nursing to see if the benefits outweigh the risks.

THE BOTTOM LINE

In some cases you can stay away from asthma-inducing irritants, such as cigarette smoke, pollen, dust mites, and pet dander. There are also lifestyle changes that can affect the severity of your asthma. Try to maintain a healthy weight and get plenty of exercise. (These are good suggestions for a healthy life, anyway.)

Everyone has different triggers and it is important to identify what causes your asthma attack. Also, the medications that are right for you may not be appropriate for your friend. Do not share medications!

Some of the side effects of these medications can get in the way of your schoolwork because they affect your concentration level. It is important to let your teachers know if you have asthma and the possible side effects of any medication you are taking.

Some medications are used preventively and others are used during an attack. Your doctor is the best source of information about which medications to take when. The doctor may prescribe more than one medication to be taken at the same time depending upon the nature of your asthma. Make sure you know the differences between relievers and preventers.

Xolair® was approved in 2003 by The Food and Drug Administration. It is estimated that it could cost as much as $10,000 per year per patient for an injection once or twice a month. Insurance will cover it in some cases, so check with your doctor and your insurance policy to see if it is right for you.

Asthma can be a life-threatening illness. While there are many potentially harmful side effects associated with these medications, the good they do must be weighed against those possibilities. The risk of uncontrolled asthma may be greater than the risk of the side effects of the medication.

It may be embarrassing for you to take your asthma medication in front of your friends. If so, talk with your doctor to see if there is something else you can take in the morning or at night so you don't have to take it at school.

Just because there are "quick-fix" medications when you are having an attack, don't stop taking your preventative medication. The complications can be very serious if you don't follow your doctor's instructions about when to take your medication.

Asthma doesn't have to keep you from doing what you love to do if you enjoy sports. There are many athletes with asthma who live and compete successfully. Learn what you need to do to make sports-related activities safe if you have exercise-induced asthma.

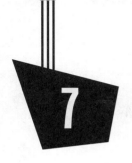

Depression

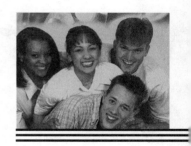

Depression is an illness that affects your body, mood, and thoughts. The three major types of depression are major depression, dysthymic depression (a less severe type of depression which is not as disabling), and bipolar disorder. Untreated, all of them interfere, in some way, with eating, sleeping, working, studying, and enjoying life.

THE MOST COMMON PRESCRIPTION MEDICATIONS

Major and Dysthymic Depression

Selective Serotonin Reuptake Inhibitors (SSRIs)

Citalopram (Celexa®)

Fluvoxamine (Luvox®)

Fluoxetine (Prozac®)

Paroxetine (Paxil®)

Sertraline (Zoloft®)

Tricyclic Antidepressants (TCAs)

Imipramine (Tofranil®)

Amitriptyline (Elavil®)

Nortriptyline (Pamelor®)

Desipramine (Norpramine®)

Monoamine Oxidase Inhibitors (MAOIs)

Phenelzine (Nardil®)

Tranylcypromine (Parnate®)

Atypical Antidepressants

Trazodone (Desyrel®)

Venlafaxine (Effexor®)

Nefazadone (Serzone®)

Mirtazapine (Remeron®)

Bupropion (Wellbutrin®)

Bipolar Disorder

Mood Stabilizers

Lithium (Eskalith®)

Carbamazepine (Tegretol®)

Valproic Acid (Depakene®)

Lamotrigine (Lamictal®)

Gabapentin (Neurontin®)

Tiagabine (Gabitril®)

Topiramate (Topamax®)

The first antidepressants were discovered because a drug for tuberculosis was observed to have unwanted, serious mental disturbances as a side effect. In the 1950s a Swiss pharmacologist, Albert Zeller, followed up on this and discovered that the drug iproniazid blocked the action of the MAO enzyme, thereby keeping it from destroying a neurotransmitter that is needed to maintain serenity. The drug was tried on severely depressed patients and it was observed to elevate their mood. This drug is no longer used for depression because it also caused liver damage, but it showed how MAOIs (Monoamine Oxidase Inhibitors) could be used as antidepressants.

Adapted from Alfred Burger, *Drugs and People, Medications, Their History and Origins, and the Way They Act* (Charlottesville: University Press of Virginia, 1986).

GENERAL INFORMATION ABOUT
HOW THESE DRUGS WORK

Severe or prolonged depression is thought to be the result of biochemical imbalances in your brain. Certain neurotransmitters regulate mood and send messages between the nerve cells in your brain. When they are not available or when there is not enough of the neurotransmitter in your brain, depression can result. This balance can be upset for genetic reasons or can happen as a result of something in your life or changing hormone levels. Medications for depression are designed to improve the balance and efficiency of the neurotransmitters in your brain.

Medications do not cure depression, but they can control the symptoms. Recent research suggests that some antidepressants may cause long-term changes in the way the nerve endings work.

SSRIs keep the neurotransmitter serotonin from being absorbed by your cells and keep it in the spaces surrounding the nerve endings of the cells in your brain. That way, the action of the serotonin is increased, which helps improve your mood.

Tricyclic antidepressants affect the levels of the neurotransmitters norepinephrine and serotonin. These neurotransmitters are linked to mood, emotion, and mental state. The antidepressants block the passage of these chemicals as they go in and out of the nerve endings and this produces a sedative effect and can elevate mood. It is possible that these medications change the way your nerve endings function over time.

MAOIs block the action of monoamine oxidase, an enzyme in your body that breaks down certain hormones. This allows the amount of the hormones to increase and provides a therapeutic effect.

The exact way the atypical antidepressants (those that don't fit well into any other medication category) work is not fully understood at this time. It is thought that they balance the levels of certain neurotransmitters, such as serotonin, norepinephrine, and dopamine, which are linked to mood, emotion, and mental state.

The way the mood stabilizers work is also not fully understood. It is thought that they interfere with the reuptake (absorption) of certain neurotransmitters and affect the way the nerves communicate with each other. They allow more of the neurotransmitters to remain in your brain so that they are more available to reduce depressive and manic episodes. The increased amount of neurotransmitter available can also have a stabilizing effect on your mood.

THE MOST COMMON POSSIBLE SIDE EFFECTS

SSRIs

- Headache
- Anxiety
- Nervousness
- Sleeplessness
- Drowsiness
- Tiredness
- Weakness
- Changes in sex drive
- Tremors
- Sweating
- Appetite loss
- Nausea
- Diarrhea
- Skin rash
- Itching

TCAs

- Blurred vision
- Dry mouth
- Dizziness or lightheadedness
- Constipation
- Difficulty urinating

◎ Sensitivity to bright light

◎ Weight changes

◎ Drowsiness

◎ Headache

◎ Increased appetite

◎ Nausea

◎ Unpleasant taste in the mouth

MAOIs

◎ Dizziness or lightheadedness (especially standing from lying or sitting)

◎ Headache

◎ Tremors

◎ Muscle twitching

◎ Sleeplessness

◎ Weakness

◎ Restlessness

◎ Drowsiness

◎ Nausea

◎ Weight changes

◎ Sexual difficulties

◎ Appetite changes (including craving for sweets)

Atypical Antidepressants

◎ Constipation

◎ Bad taste in the mouth

◎ Nausea

◎ Vomiting

◎ Blood pressure changes

◎ Dizziness

◎ Confusion

◎ Drowsiness

◎ Fatigue

- Lightheadedness
- Sleeplessness
- Agitation
- Blurred vision
- Sexual problems
- Dry mouth
- Headache
- Tremors
- Weakness
- Increased sweating
- Loss of appetite

Mood Stabilizers

- Drowsiness
- Dizziness
- Unusual tiredness or weakness
- Abnormal eye movements or twitching
- Vision problems
- Skin rash
- Nausea
- Vomiting
- Indigestion
- Unusual weight changes
- Loss of appetite
- Tremors
- Diarrhea
- Hair loss
- Unsteadiness

OTHER PRECAUTIONS

SSRIs

- There has been a lot of controversy concerning prescribing these medications for patients under the age of eighteen.

Work closely with your doctor if SSRIs have been prescribed for you.

◎ Do not stop taking antidepressants without talking with your doctor. Some of them have side effects that occur if you stop abruptly and you may need to taper off the medication.

◎ These medications have been known to affect pregnancies and can pass into breast milk. Check with your doctor if you are pregnant or nursing.

◎ These medications can add to the effects of alcohol and other central nervous system depressants.

◎ These medications can make you drowsy. Make sure you know how they affect you before you do anything that requires your full alertness, like driving.

TCAs

◎ Smoking and oral contraceptives may reduce the effects of TCAs.

◎ These medications can add to the effects of alcohol and other central nervous system depressants.

◎ These medications have been known to affect pregnancies and can pass into breast milk. Check with your doctor if you are pregnant or nursing.

◎ These medications can make your skin more sensitive to the sun. Make sure you take proper precautions when in the sun and avoid tanning booths and sun lamps.

MAOIs

◎ MAOIs are rarely used in children because of the restrictions to what you can eat. When taking MAOIs, you need to avoid certain foods like pickles, many cheeses and wine, and decongestant medication due to the risk of an increase in blood pressure from the interaction of the tyramine in the food and the MAO inhibitors. You may need to be on a special diet if you are taking MAOIs.

◎ You should not take MAOIs and other types of medications, especially those that increase the activity of serotonin, together or within a certain time period.

⊚ These medications can add to the effects of alcohol and other central nervous system depressants and could cause serious side effects.

Atypical Antidepressants

⊚ These medications can make you drowsy. Make sure you know how they affect you before you do anything that requires your full alertness.

⊚ These medications can add to the effects of alcohol and other central nervous system depressants.

⊚ These medications have been known to affect pregnancies and can pass into breast milk. Check with your doctor if you are pregnant or nursing.

⊚ Do not take these medications at or near the same time as you take MAOIs.

⊚ Serzone®, an atypical antidepressant that is not included in this list, has been taken off the market in the United States and other countries because of the risk of liver failure. Make sure you monitor this if Serzone® is working for you.

Mood Stabilizers

⊚ These medications can add to the effects of alcohol and other central nervous system depressants.

⊚ These medications have been known to affect pregnancies and can pass into breast milk. Check with your doctor if you are pregnant or nursing.

THE BOTTOM LINE

Sometimes you have to try a variety of medications before you hit on the right one. Don't give up if the first one doesn't work for you. Also, many of the medications take a while before they begin to work. Again, don't give up if you don't feel better immediately. Give it the amount of time that the doctor recommends before you look for something else.

Not all depression is the same and a medication that works

for your friend may not be the right one for you. Many of the medications are not federally approved for teens, but your doctor can prescribe them if he or she thinks it is the right one for you and follows you closely while you are taking it. Do not take any medication for feelings of depression without the advice of your doctor.

Many of these medications are used in combination with others and many cannot be combined. Your doctor knows which medications work well together and which don't.

Some of the medications must be stopped gradually. Do not stop taking any medication without discussing it with your doctor and finding out how to taper off safely.

The risks of not taking medication for depression can be greater than the side effects of the medications, especially if you

I take medication for bipolar disorder four times a day, two doses at school. I take them at lunch and right after school. The pills make me really sleepy during the day at school, but I have only been taking them since April. Sometimes I fall asleep in class. The teachers know that I am going through trials of medication and that there may be side effects, but they don't really notice when I fall asleep because they haven't woken me up. I did pretty bad on some tests because I missed things in class, but I did get 100 on a math quiz. The doctor thinks the sleepiness will wear off. Most of my friends already know I take meds so they don't ask where I'm going. When I wasn't on meds, I had, like, these mood swings and now I don't have them as much. Some of my thoughts are clearer since I have been on meds. Sometimes the medications can have a good effect even if you hate taking it and feel, "I'm sick of this and don't want to take it anymore." My friend stopped taking meds for bipolar because she was sick of taking it and she's not doing too well because of that.
—Heather, 14 years old, ninth grade

have thoughts of hurting yourself or others.

Some people can be helped by talking with a "talk therapist," either with or without medication. You might want to try that first.

There has been a lot of publicity about whether Paxil or other SSRIs cause suicide. At this point, doctors don't know whether it is the result of the medications or is the result of the condition. However, it should make you more alert to questions about the medication you are using. A good working relationship with your doctor is especially important when you are on medications for depression.

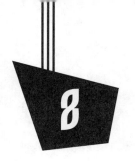

Diabetes

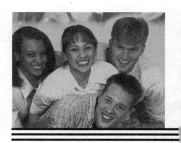

Type 1 or juvenile diabetes is the inability of your pancreas to make and use insulin. Without insulin, glucose (the main fuel for your body) cannot get into your cells in order for you to have the energy you need to stay alive. Without insulin, the glucose stays in your blood and passes out of your body with urine. With type 2 diabetes, the pancreas is usually producing enough insulin, but the body cannot use it effectively. Type 2 diabetes is relatively rare in teens and is usually the result of lifestyle problems.

THE MOST COMMON PRESCRIPTION MEDICATIONS

Insulin—For Type 1 and Type 2

- Quick acting—Acts within five to fifteen minutes and lasts three to four hours:

  Lispro (Humalog®)

  Aspart (NovoLog®)

- Short acting—Acts in thirty minutes and lasts five to eight hours:

  Insulin Regular (Humulin R®)

- Intermediate acting—Acts in one to three hours and lasts sixteen to twenty-four hours:

  NPH Insulin (Humulin N®)

  Lente Insulin (Humulin L®)

- Long acting—Acts in four to six hours and lasts twenty-four to twenty-eight hours:

  Ultralente Insulin (Humulin U®)

◎ **Peakless—Acts for twenty-four hours:**

Glargine (Lantus®)

◎ **Intermediate- and short-acting mixtures—Acts in thirty minutes and lasts sixteen to twenty-four hours:**

NPH Insulin and Insulin (Humulin 50/50®)

Pills—For Type 2

Biguanides

Metformin (Glucophage®)

Thiazolidinediones (Glitazones)

Rosiglitazone (Avandia®)

Pioglitazone (Actos®)

Alpha-Glucosidase Inhibitors

Acarbose (Precose®)

Miglitol (Glyset®)

GENERAL INFORMATION ABOUT HOW THESE DRUGS WORK

If you have type 1 diabetes it is because your immune system attacked and destroyed the beta cells in your pancreas that produce insulin. The insulin levels in your blood drop, and glucose can no longer enter the cells in your body to be used as energy. The goal of any treatment is to keep your glucose levels as close to normal as possible.

Insulin is a hormone that is taken by injection (shot) and lowers your blood glucose by causing glucose (sugar) to move from the blood into the cells of your body. Insulin does not cure diabetes. Insulin is injected because if it is taken by mouth it is destroyed by stomach acid. The amount of insulin you need is determined by your diet and the amount of exercise you engage in.

Diabetes pills for type 2 can only work if your pancreas is creating some insulin. They are not a substitute for insulin. For teens, they are also not a substitute for lifestyle changes. Exercise and healthy eating habits are the first line of treatment for type 2 diabetes in teens. There are pills that are prescribed for teens whose diabetes needs more aggressive treatment.

Biguanides lower the amount of glucose made by your liver.

Thiazolidinedione makes your body more sensitive to the insulin and makes the insulin work better. It reduces the amount of sugar produced by the liver and increases the amount of sugar used by your liver, muscles, and fat cells.

Alpha-glucosidase inhibitors slow and block the breakdown and absorption of the starches you eat and therefore slow the rise of your blood sugar levels.

THE MOST COMMON POSSIBLE SIDE EFFECTS

Insulin

- Cold sweats
- Rapid heartbeat
- Hunger
- Headache
- Shakiness
- Weight gain
- Anxiety or nervousness

Biguanide

- Diarrhea
- Nausea
- Vomiting
- Abdominal bloating
- Excess gas
- Loss of appetite

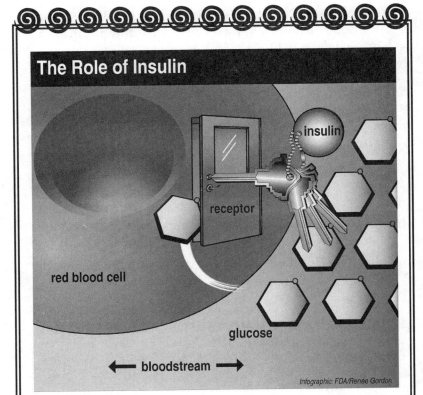

The Role of Insulin

The Role of Insulin

Carbohydrates that we eat make our blood glucose (sugar) rise. To utilize the carbohydrates and lower the blood sugar, insulin opens the doors of the body's cells to glucose circulating in the blood. The glucose enters the cells and is used as the cells' fuel for energy. Insulin binds to a spot on the cell surface called a receptor. Likened to a lock and key, insulin is the key that opens up the lock (receptor) so that glucose can pass through the door into the cell. Using this analogy in type 1 diabetes, the keys have been stolen (no insulin is made by the pancreas). In type 2, the door won't open fully even with the right key (insulin resistance). Christopher D. Saudek, Richard R. Rubin, and Cynthia S. Shump, *The Johns Hopkins Guide to Diabetes* (Baltimore: Johns Hopkins University Press, 1997).

Reprinted with permission from the Food and Drug Administration.

Thiazolidinedione

- Upper respiratory tract infection
- Headache
- Sinus problems
- Muscle aches
- Tooth problems
- Sore throat
- Liver abnormalities

Alpha-Glucosidase Inhibitors

- Stomach gas (flatulence)
- Abdominal pain
- Diarrhea

OTHER PRECAUTIONS

Insulin

- Insulin does not seem to affect pregnancy or breast-feeding, but both pregnancy and breast-feeding can affect your insulin requirements. Work closely with your doctor if you have or are planning to have children.
- It is recommended that insulin be the drug of choice if you are pregnant or breast-feeding.

Biguanide

- Combining this medication with alcohol can cause severe low blood sugar.

Thiazolidinedione

- Thiazolidinediones may make birth control pills less effective.
- This type of medication may cause you to gain weight.
- Combining this medication with alcohol can cause severe low blood sugar.

Alpha-Glucosidase Inhibitors

◎ **Combining this medication with alcohol can cause severe low blood sugar.**

THE BOTTOM LINE

Although there are many side effects associated with the medications for diabetes, there is a greater danger if you do not take the medications and maintain a healthy diet and exercise program. The medications, diet, and exercise enable you to keep your blood sugar at a healthy level. If your blood sugar stays too high, the major complications of diabetes are heart disease, blood vessel disease, blindness, kidney damage, high blood pressure, gum disease, and nerve problems. If your blood sugar level is too low, you might feel weak or dizzy and notice changes in your heartbeat. In serious cases, you could pass out or have a seizure.

Your diabetes medications and other medications you take can cause a drop in your blood sugar levels. You should always carry an emergency supply of things like hard candy or glucose tablets for low blood sugar.

Healthy eating and physical activity are important in the treatment of diabetes. Insulin and pills can't do it alone. You need to make sure you eat a healthy diet because the foods you eat affect your blood glucose levels. You won't always be able to go along with the crowd at meal times and eat at irregular times like many teenagers like to do. You also may need to change your diet if your glucose levels are too high or too low.

If you are taking insulin or pills, you have increased risk of low blood sugar and other side effects if you drink alcohol. You need to weigh that risk with your need to drink and be part of the crowd. Not all people with diabetes need to stay away from alcohol completely. Discuss this with your doctor to see what is right for you.

There can be an increase in the blood sugar lowering effect of all of the type 2 medications if you take sulfa drugs, aspirin, or other nonsteroidal anti-inflammatory drugs. This can also occur if you don't eat enough, or exercise properly, or don't have enough food in you.

Exercise, along with the proper foods, helps keep your weight at the right level. Exercise also helps the insulin work better to lower your blood glucose. Your exercise program may not be the same as your friends', because certain types of exercise, like weight lifting, may not be good for you if you have high blood pressure. Check with your doctor about the best exercise program for you and stick with it.

Vigilance is also important. Glucose levels must be monitored many times daily to keep the levels from going too high or too low.

There are many things that you do or eat that can affect the amount and time you need to take your medications. Colds, bacterial infections, and stress can change your blood sugar levels and your needs for insulin. You need to keep your doctor informed of any changes in your life or lifestyle to avoid major problems.

You need to have a close working relationship with your doctor to make sure that you get all the care you need. You might also need to work with a dietician and a personal trainer. Make sure your health care providers are people you respect and can be honest and upfront with.

All of these medications interact in some way with other medications you might be taking. Make sure you tell your doctor about any other medications and alternative remedies you are using. Also, make sure that the life of the medication has not expired.

You also need to work closely with the nurse at your school. You will be in school for a major part of each day and the nurse needs to know what to do to help you maintain your levels as well as be aware if complications arise. You can help set up a medical management plan or school health plan to be kept on file at the school for maintenance and emergencies.

You should wear a medical ID tag when you are away from home. In an emergency, if you are not able to tell someone about your diabetes condition and the medications you are taking, the tag will make sure you get the care you need.

I used to take Lantus insulin. You have to take insulin by a huge shot at the beginning on the day. It really hurt. Then I took a fast-acting insulin through a shot. I had to give them to myself and I hated the shots. I had to take them every time I ate something. Now I take a fast-acting insulin through a pump and it is so much better. The insulin comes in a cartridge that I wear on my belt loop. It looks like a beeper and a lot of people mistake it for a beeper. I just press in the amount I want. It is like giving myself a shot without doing anything. It is so much easier to manage and you have more control of how much insulin you give yourself and your blood sugar will be more normal.

The insulin goes into a catheter on my stomach or hip. It can go anywhere, but I like it on the stomach or hip the best. I have to change the catheter every 2 days. I use a numbing cream and let it sit for about thirty minutes before I change the catheter. Otherwise it really hurts. My friend has a pump too and it is nice to have someone else who has it.

I play a lot of sports—soccer, basketball, volleyball, track, and cross country—so I am usually away from home when I need to change my catheter. The catheter doesn't interfere with the sports, but I usually take the pump off when I am playing. I am allowed to take it off for an hour at a time. It is always giving you a little insulin, but it is ok to miss one hour.

There are not side effects from the insulin, but there can be problems when I have taken too much or too little. I don't always know the amount of carbs in what I eat so I am not always putting in the right amount. When my blood sugar gets too low, I must eat something really fast. I can feel it happening. I feel really crappy and it is not fun. When I don't give myself enough, I get really high. Then I get angry and mean.

The bad thing with the pump is that the catheter can come out and you don't realize it until you have the side effect. Then I have to do the whole set change and it takes about thirty minutes to one hour. It is not usually a hassle.

At first, I didn't want to take my blood sugar. I thought if I felt fine then I was fine. My advice is to test your blood sugar any time you are doing something different.—Laura Kate, eighth grade

Your body changes as you get older and, even if you do everything right, your diabetes may be harder to control as your hormone levels change. Find someone to talk to about how you are feeling.

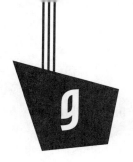

Eating Disorders

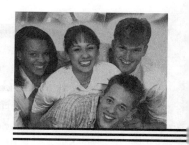

Eating disorders are extreme and unhealthy emotional, behavioral, and psychological attitudes about food and body weight. The main eating disorders are anorexia nervosa, or anorexia, bulimia nervosa, or bulimia, and binge eating disorder, BED. Anorexia nervosa is an intense fear of being fat so that you hardly eat at all. Bulimia nervosa is also an intense fear of being fat, but you eat large amounts of food and then get rid of it by vomiting (purging) or taking laxatives. BED is repeated episodes of compulsive overeating without purging.

THE MOST COMMON PRESCRIPTION MEDICATIONS

Selective Serotonin Reuptake Inhibitors (SSRIs)

Citalopram (Celexa®)

Fluoxetine (Prozac®)

Fluvoxamine (Luvox®)

Paroxetine (Paxil®)

Sertraline (Zoloft®)

GENERAL INFORMATION ABOUT HOW THESE DRUGS WORK

Eating disorders arise from a variety of behavioral, emotional, social, and psychological reasons. There is some reason to believe that a chemical reaction in the brain is involved in an eating disorder. Also, since depression and anxiety are often associated with the eating disorder, it lends further credibility to the theory of the chemical imbalance in the brain. Therefore, medications for the disorders are those that treat the underlying depression and anxiety by regulating the neurotransmitters in the brain in order to achieve long-term results. Medications for depression, when used to treat eating disorders, are designed to improve the balance and efficiency of the neurotransmitters in your brain in order to alleviate the depression and anxiety that are associated with the eating disorder.

THE MOST COMMON POSSIBLE SIDE EFFECTS

SSRIs

- Headache
- Anxiety
- Nervousness
- Sleeplessness
- Drowsiness
- Tiredness
- Weakness
- Changes in sex drive
- Tremors
- Sweating
- Appetite loss
- Nausea
- Diarrhea
- Skin rash
- Itching

OTHER PRECAUTIONS

SSRIs

- There has been a lot of controversy concerning prescribing these medications for patients under the age of eighteen. Work closely with your doctor if SSRIs have been prescribed for you.

- Do not stop taking antidepressants without talking with your doctor. Some of them have side effects that occur if you stop abruptly and you may need to taper off the medication.

- These medications have been known to affect pregnancies and can pass into breast milk. Check with your doctor if you are pregnant or nursing.

- These medications can add to the effects of alcohol and other central nervous system depressants.

- These medications can make you drowsy. Make sure you know how they affect you before you do anything that requires your full alertness.

THE BOTTOM LINE

According to the National Institute of Mental Health, the first line of treatment is psychological services and nutritional rehabilitation. The sooner these disorders are diagnosed and treated, the better the chances for a positive outcome. Eating disorders are complex and the management requires a comprehensive treatment plan. It is important to keep in mind that eating disorders can be treated and a healthy weight can be restored.

In some cases, it is necessary to stay in the hospital until a normal weight is achieved.

It may be necessary to get your weight to a normal limit before taking certain of the medications to treat the underlying depression.

There has been a lot of publicity about whether Paxil or other SSRIs cause suicide. At this point, doctors don't know whether it is the result of the medications or the result of the condition, however it should make you more alert to the medications you are using. A good working relationship with your doctor is especially important when you are on medications for eating disorders.

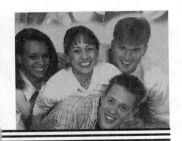

Eczema

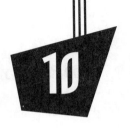

Eczema is a group of skin conditions that range from hot, dry, itchy skin to broken, raw, bleeding skin.

THE MOST COMMON PRESCRIPTION MEDICATIONS

Topical Immunomodulators (TIMs)

Tacrolimus (Protopic®)

Pimecrolimus (Elidel Cream®)

Oral Corticosteroids

Hydrocortisone (Hydrocortone®)

Methylprednisolone (Medrol®)

Prednisolone (Prelone®)

Prednisone (Deltasone®)

Topical Corticosteroid

Low Potency

Hydrocortisone (Dermacort®)

Desonide (DesOwen®)

Triamcinolone (Aristocort®)

Midpotency

Flurandrenolide (Cordan®)

Mometasone (Elocon®)

High Potency

Fluocinonide (Lidex®)

Betamethasone (Diprolene®)

Very High Potency

Clobetasol Propionate (Cormax®)

Over-the-Counter Lubricants

Multiple varieties and brand names

GENERAL INFORMATION ABOUT
HOW THESE DRUGS WORK

Doctors are not exactly sure what causes eczema and there is no known cure at this time. There is some thought (and research) supporting the idea that an immune system imbalance is, at least, partially involved. The medications and treatments help to heal the skin and keep it healthy, treat flare-ups, and minimize the symptoms when they occur.

TIMs act on the skin cells and alter the cells' reaction to the inflammation. They suppress the immune system by blocking the action of the cells.

Corticosteroid creams reduce the inflammation during flare-ups of the eczema by interfering with your body's ability to produce inflammation.

Oral corticosteroids block the release of chemicals in the body that produce inflammation and suppress the activity of your immune system.

Over-the-counter lubricants work by providing a seal over your skin to reduce water loss and therefore the dryness associated with the loss of moisture on the skin. This is the first line of defense against eczema. They should be used often but especially immediately after bathing. They should be as free from fragrance and chemicals as possible. Creams and ointments work better because they have less alcohol and last longer on your skin.

THE MOST COMMON POSSIBLE SIDE EFFECTS

TIMs

- Burning, stinging, itching, or redness at site of application

Oral Corticosteroids

- Short term:
  - Fluid retention and weight gain
  - Slow healing of wounds
  - Easy bruising
  - Increased appetite
  - Indigestion
- Long term:
  - Slow growth
  - Lowered resistance to infections
  - Eye problems (including cataracts)
  - Headache
  - Muscle weakness
  - Unusual increase in facial hair growth
  - Menstruation problems
  - Thinning skin

Topical Corticosteroid

- Burning
- Itching
- Irritation
- Acne
- Dry and cracking skin

OTHER PRECAUTIONS

TIMs

- These medications can make your skin more sensitive to the sun. Make sure you take proper precautions when in the sun and avoid tanning booths and sun lamps.

Oral Corticosteroids

◎ Corticosteroids should not be stopped without supervision from your doctor. Abruptly stopping this type of medication can have serious side effects.

◎ Because long-term use of corticosteroids lowers your resistance to infections, check with your doctor before having a vaccination or before making plans to be with others who have been vaccinated.

◎ Oral contraceptives may also increase the side effects of corticosteroids.

◎ These medications have been known to affect pregnancies and can pass into breast milk. Check with your doctor if you are pregnant or nursing.

Topical Corticosteroid

◎ There are many types and strengths of steroid creams. Do not share medications with anyone as the cream prescribed for your friend may make your eczema worse or cause other unwanted side effects.

THE BOTTOM LINE

Complimentary treatments, such as Evening Primrose oil, have been used by some people to treat eczema. The complimentary treatments have not been researched or approved for this condition. It is important to discuss any alternative treatments with your doctor, as there could be interactional side effects with the medications you are taking.

It is very important not to scratch your eczema, but that is probably the one thing you want to do when it flares up. Keep an emollient handy to spread on when you feel the urge to scratch. If you MUST scratch, be very careful not to damage your skin further.

You will need to develop a routine to help you control the itching. This will be personal to you and your lifestyle and might involve how often you bathe, the type of soap you use, when to apply emollients, the type of heat in your house, the fabric of the clothes you wear, and other medications or remedies you use.

Antihistamines can reduce inflammation during flare-ups, reduce nighttime scratching, and allow you to get more sleep. Check them out in the allergies chapter and talk with your doctor about whether they might help you.

In severe flare-ups, it is possible for your skin to become infected. In that case, your doctor may also prescribe an antibiotic. Check the chapter on inflammatory bowel disease for information on side effects associated with antibiotics.

It is important to let your school know if you have eczema, as you may need accommodations for maintenance of your medications. Some possible accommodations are:

- **Keeping an emollient in a comfortable place and ability to leave the classroom to apply it as needed.**
- **Having a flexible schedule if oral medications cause you to be extremely drowsy in the mornings.**

Ultraviolet light therapy has been successful in controlling the symptoms of some types of eczema. Check with your doctor to see if this might be helpful for you.

11 Inflammatory Bowel Disease (IBD)

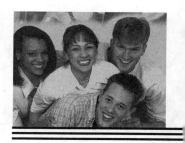

Inflammatory bowel diseases are ulcerative colitis and Crohn's disease, which cause chronic abdominal pain, intermittent, severe diarrhea, and weight or growth problems.

THE MOST COMMON PRESCRIPTION MEDICATIONS

Anti-Inflammatory Drugs

Corticosteroids

Prednisone (Deltasone®)

Methylprednisolone (Medrol®)

Aminosalicylates (5-aminosalicylic acid or 5-ASA)

Mesalamine (Asacol®)

Balsalazide (Colazal®)

Sulfasalazine (Azulfidine®)

Antibiotics

Metronidazole (Flagyl®)

Ciprofloxacin (Cipro®)

Immunosuppressants

Azathioprine (Imuran®)

Cyclosporine (Sandimmune®)

> [F]rom the beginning of 1938 to the end of 1940, stomach and
> colon problems continued to plague him (John F. Kennedy). In
> February 1938, he (John F. Kennedy) had gone back to the Mayo
> Clinic for more study. The Mayo treatment for ulcerated colitis
> now consisted of blood transfusions, liver extract, nicotinic
> acid, thiamine chloride, and Neoprontosil, a sulphur drug, but
> the clinic itself acknowledged that its therapy was of limited
> value.
>
>   Robert Dallek, *An Unfinished Life, John F. Kennedy 1917-
> 1963* (Boston: Little Brown and Company, 2003), 80.

Mercaptopurine or 6-MP (Purinethol®)

Methotrexate (Rheumatrex®)

Biologic Response Modifiers (BRMs)

Infliximab (Remicade®)

GENERAL INFORMATION ABOUT HOW THESE DRUGS WORK

It is thought that inflammatory bowel disease is partially related
to a problem with the immune system. Your immune system
consists of immune cells and the proteins they produce. Together
they protect your body against harmful invasions. They do this
by inflaming the tissues where the invasion occurs. Normally, this
happens only when there is the presence of a foreign, harmful
invasion. With IBD, the immune system does not turn off and is
chronically activated, even without the presence of a foreign
invasion. The diseases cause the walls of the large and/or small
intestines to become inflamed. When this happens, the lining of
the intestinal wall gets red and swells. It often becomes irritated
and could bleed and prevent the intestines from properly
absorbing nutrients from the food you eat. This inflammation
damages the intestines. There is no cure but medications can help
control the symptoms and medications are being developed to
help regulate the immune system.

Corticosteroids block the release of chemicals in the body that produce inflammation and suppress the activity of your immune system.

It is not clear how aminosalicylates work. It is thought they work directly in the colon and inhibit inflammation. These medications have been modified chemically so they are not absorbed by your stomach or upper intestines. They can reach your ileum and colon and the active ingredient is released there and is available to treat the inflammation. Balsalazide appears to work in the colon by blocking chemicals that cause the bowel to be overactive and inflamed.

Antibiotics destroy bacteria by blocking some of their cell functions, which interferes with their growth and causes them to die. This contributes to the healing of the damage to the colon.

Immunosuppressants target cells that grow at a fast rate and are able to block the action of some immune cells and interfere with the action of other immune cells that cause inflammation.

BRMs are given by injection. They block the action of proteins that can promote inflammation and pain. They bind to the protein, acting like a sponge, and keep it from the joints and blood. They combine with an essential component in the inflammatory process, rendering the cell inactive.

THE MOST COMMON POSSIBLE SIDE EFFECTS

Corticosteroids

- Short term:
  - Fluid retention and weight gain
  - Slow healing of wounds
  - Easy bruising
  - Increased appetite
  - Indigestion
  - Insomnia
- Long term:
  - Slow growth
  - Lowered resistance to infections

Physicians in the 1930s and 1940s did not realize what today is common medical knowledge: namely, that adrenal extracts (corticosteroids, or anti-inflammatory agents) are effective in treating acute ulcerative colitis but can have deleterious long-term chronic effects, including osteoporosis with vertebral column deterioration and peptic ulcers.
Robert Dallek, *An Unfinished Life, John F. Kennedy 1917–1963* (Boston: Little Brown and Company, 2003), 76.

- Eye problems (including cataracts)
- Headache
- Muscle weakness
- Unusual increase in facial hair growth
- Menstruation problems
- Thinning skin

Aminosalicylates

- Abdominal pain, cramps, or discomfort
- Generalized pain
- Stomach rumbling
- For Sulfasalazine, in addition:
  - Headache
  - Itching
  - Skin rash
  - Skin sensitivity to sunlight

- Nausea
- Vomiting
- Loss of appetite

Antibiotics

- Nausea
- Headache
- Dizziness
- Vomiting
- Diarrhea
- Stomach cramps

Immunosuppressants

- Nausea
- Vomiting
- Loss of appetite
- Increased hair growth on body and face or hair loss
- Mouth sores or swollen and bleeding gums
- High blood pressure
- Hand tremors
- Kidney problems
- Reduced white blood counts
- Hair loss

BRMs

- Headache
- Nausea
- Cold symptoms
- Abdominal pain
- Unusual tiredness
- Fever
- Vomiting

OTHER PRECAUTIONS

Corticosteroids

- Corticosteroids should not be stopped without supervision from your doctor. Abruptly stopping this type of medication can have serious side effects.
- Because long-term use of corticosteroids lowers your resistance to infections, check with your doctor before having a vaccination or before making plans to be with others who have been vaccinated.
- Oral contraceptives may also increase the side effects of corticosteroids.
- These medications have been known to affect pregnancies and can pass into breast milk. Check with your doctor if you are pregnant or nursing.

Aminosalicylates

- These medications have been known to affect pregnancies and can pass into breast milk. Check with your doctor if you are pregnant or nursing.
- Aminosalicylates are related chemically to aspirin. If you are allergic to aspirin, you should not take these medications.
- Sulfasalazine is a sulfa drug and should not be taken if you are allergic to sulfa drugs.
- Sulfasalazine can make your skin more sensitive to the sun. Make sure you take proper precautions when in the sun and avoid tanning booths and sun lamps.
- Sulfasalazine can affect sperm count and sperm function.
- Sulfasalazine can turn your urine an orange-yellow color and may also stain contact lenses.

Antibiotics

- These medications have been known to affect pregnancies and can pass into breast milk. Check with your doctor if you are pregnant or nursing.
- Drinking alcohol can increase the side effects of these medications and can cause severe nausea, vomiting, and skin

flushing. Be sure to check that other medications you might be taking, like cough syrups, do not contain alcohol.

◎ These medications can make your skin more sensitive to the sun. Make sure you take proper precautions when in the sun and avoid tanning booths and sun lamps.

Immunosuppressants

◎ Drinking alcohol can increase the side effects of these medications. Be sure to check that other medications you might be taking, like cough syrups, do not contain alcohol.

◎ These medications suppress your immune system and may interfere with your body's ability to fight other infections while you are on it. Long-term use could lead to lymphoma and liver problems.

◎ These medications have been known to affect pregnancies and can pass into breast milk. Check with your doctor if you are pregnant or nursing.

◎ These medications can reduce sperm count and there is a higher incidence of miscarriages if the male's partner does conceive.

◎ Some immunosuppressants should absolutely not be used if you are pregnant as they can cause abortion. Check this carefully with your doctor.

BRMs

◎ BRMs are relatively new drugs and there is little information about long-term risks. Their safety during pregnancy or nursing is not known. Check with your doctor about the possible risks.

◎ These medications suppress your immune system and may interfere with your body's ability to fight other infections while you are on them.

THE BOTTOM LINE

There is no indication that the disease is caused or made worse by food (although some people find that milk, alcohol, hot spices, or fiber make their symptoms worse), so you can eat anything you want as long as it does not worsen your symptoms. Your diet should be a healthy one since the loss of nutrients is such a problem. You are in luck now that the fast food restaurants are beginning to label the nutritional value of their foods. You may want to take nutritional supplements if you are losing too many nutrients. Check with your doctor about what you may need to take.

Aminosalicylates can also be administered by enema—Rowasa®—and by suppository—Canasa®. Both have been effective when the inflammation is near the rectum.

If medications don't work, surgery may be recommended to remove the diseased part of the colon. This usually helps to free you of the disease and symptoms for a while, but many times Crohn's disease will recur. Ulcerative colitis is often cured by the surgery.

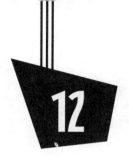

Juvenile Rheumatoid Arthritis (JRA)

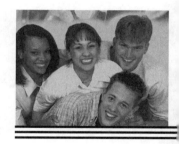

Juvenile Rheumatoid Arthritis (JRA) is an inflammation or stiffness of a joint or joints that affects children under age sixteen. There are different types of JRA depending upon how many joints are involved and whether internal organs are involved.

THE MOST COMMON MEDICATIONS

Over-the-Counter—Nonsteroidal Anti-Inflammatory Drugs (NSAIDs)

Ibuprofen (Advil®)

Naproxen (Aleve®)

Aspirin (Arthritis Pain Formula®)

Choline salicylate (Arthropan®)

Prescription—Nonsteroidal Anti-Inflammatory Drugs (NSAIDs)

Diclofenac (Voltaren®)

Tolmetin (Tolectin®)

Choline and Magnesium salicylate (Tricosal®)

Prescription COX-2 Inhibitors

Celecoxib (Celebrex®)

Valdecoxib (Bextra®)

Analgesics

Over-the-Counter Analgesics

Acetaminophen (Tylenol®)

Prescription Analgesics with Acetaminophen

Acetaminophen/Codeine (Tylenol with Codeine®)

Hydrocodone/Acetaminophen (Vicodin®)

Oxycodone/Acetaminophen (Percocet®)

Tramadol/Acetaminophen (Ultracet®)

Over-the-Counter Topical Analgesics/Counterirritants

Capsaicin (Zostrix®)

Trolamine Salicylate (Aspercreme®)

Menthol (Eucalyptamint®)

Methyl Salicylate (BenGay®)

Methyl Salicylate and Menthol (IcyHot®)

Prescription Disease-Modifying Antirheumatic Drugs (DMARDs)

Gold (Myochrisine®)

Hydroxychloroquine (Plaquenil®)

Leflunomide (Arava®)

Methotrexate (Rheumatrex®)

Sulfasalazine (Azulfidine®)

Prescription Immunosuppressants

Azothiaprine (Imuran®)

d-Penicillamine (Cuprimine®)

Cyclosporine (Sandimmune®)

Prescription Corticosteroids

Prednisone (Deltasone®)

A Greek doctor during the first-century used "oxymel," a sour honey to treat arthritis. Early Europeans suggested increasing sweating to expel toxins from the body. Other European peasants used poultices of white cabbage leaves and French villagers used poultices of buttercups applied to the area of pain.

Dian Dincin Buchman, *Ancient Healing Secrets* (New York: Random House, 1996).

Prescription Biologic Response Modifiers (BRMs)

Etanercept (Enbrel®)

Adalimumab (Humira®)

Infliximab (Remicade®)

GENERAL INFORMATION ABOUT HOW THESE DRUGS WORK

JRA occurs when your immune system (white blood cells) releases chemicals that attack healthy cells and tissues instead of fighting off harmful viruses and bacteria as it is supposed to do. This accumulation of white cells results in the promotion of tissue damage. When this happens inflammation and the pain associated with the inflammation occur. Chronic inflammation results in the loss of cartilage and the formation of scar tissue that leads to filling of the joint spaces and the loss of joint motion. The main goals of treatment focus on quality of life—helping you maintain a good level of physical and social activity. The medications work by reducing inflammation, relieving pain, and preventing complications.

NSAIDs work by blocking your body's production of specific hormones and chemicals that contribute to inflammation and pain. The OTC medications control pain. NSAIDS can control inflammation. The prescriptive dose also controls the underlying inflammation.

COX-2 inhibitors are NSAIDs that do not block the hormone that helps maintain the protective lining in your stomach.

> While antifever drugs were being discovered and put to use, the most familiar of all, aspirin (acetylsalicylic acid), was lying unappreciated on a chemist's shelf. In 1838, salicyclic acid was manufactured from salicin, an ingredient of willow bark and used to relieve fever and rheumatic pain. Fifteen years later, a relative of salicin, acetylsalicyclic acid, was synthesized by the German chemist Charles Gerhardt. Only in the 1890s, however, was this compound checked for antirheumatic effects. The Bayer laboratories in Elberfield (Germany) first tested animals, then arranged for clinical trials. Their work, published in 1899, showed that the compound was indeed effective in controlling pain and inflammation both in rheumatism and other conditions, and in reducing fever as well. Bayer patented the production process and named the new drug Aspirin.
>
> Roy Porter, ed., *The Cambridge Illustrated History of Medicine* (Cambridge: Cambridge University Press, 1966), 26.

Analgesics are thought to control pain by lowering your pain threshold, but they do not help with inflammation. Some prescriptive analgesics contain narcotics. Tramadol is thought to reduce the uptake (absorption) of the neurotransmitters serotonin and norepinephrine into the nerves. Tramadol is not a narcotic.

Topical analgesics work by seeping through the skin and slowing the pain. They either block the transmission of pain to the brain or fool the pain by creating a feeling of cold or heat.

Disease-modifying antirheumatic drugs (DMARDs) work by suppressing the immune cells that are responsible for inflammation. These medications work slowly and are usually combined with a faster acting medication to help suppress symptoms.

> The old Greek name for pain was *algesis*, and chemicals that counteract pain are called analgesics or analgetics.
> Alfred Burger, *Drugs and People, Medications, Their History and Origins, and the Way They Act* (Charlottesville: University Press of Virginia, 1986).

Immunosuppressants target cells that grow at a fast rate and are able to block the action of some immune cells. They also interfere with the action of other immune cells that cause inflammation.

Corticosteroids can ease the inflammation of the joints and organs. They block the release of chemicals in the body that produce inflammation and suppress the activity of your immune system. They are usually used in combination with other medications for a short time until the other medications begin to work. If they are used alone, the lowest dose with the best effect is recommended.

Biologic response modifiers (BRMs) are given by injection. They block the action of proteins that can promote inflammation and pain. They bind to the protein, acting like a sponge, and keep it from the joints and blood. They combine with an essential component in the inflammatory process, rendering the cell inactive.

THE MOST COMMON POSSIBLE SIDE EFFECTS

NSAIDs

- Diarrhea
- Nausea
- Vomiting
- Stomach cramps and pain
- Gas or heartburn
- Tinnitus or ringing in the ear
- With aspirin—gastrointestinal bleeding and blood in the stool

COX-2 Inhibitors

- Headache
- Heartburn
- Gas
- Nausea
- Acid or sour stomach

- Abdominal pain
- Diarrhea
- Respiratory infection
- GI bleeding

OTC Analgesics

- Few side effects when taken as recommended
- See "other precautions" for additional warnings

Prescription Analgesics

- Nausea
- Vomiting
- Upset stomach
- Lightheadedness
- Dizziness
- Drowsiness
- Constipation
- Headache
- Itching
- Weakness
- Sweating
- Diarrhea

Topical Analgesics

- Warmth, stinging, or burning at the site of application

DMARDs

- Diarrhea
- Nausea
- Vomiting
- Headache

- Loss of appetite and weight loss
- Vision problems
- Swelling
- Stomach pain
- Hair loss
- Skin rash
- Itching
- Skin sensitivity to sunlight
- Reduced white blood count
- Mouth sores
- Chest congestion

Immunosuppressants

- Nausea
- Vomiting
- Loss of appetite
- Increased hair growth on body and face or hair loss
- Mouth sores or swollen and bleeding gums
- High blood pressure
- Hand tremors
- Kidney problems

Corticosteroids

- Short term:
    - Fluid retention and weight gain
    - Slow healing of wounds
    - Easy bruising
    - Increased appetite
    - Indigestion
    - Insomnia
- Long term:
    - Slow growth
    - Lowered resistance to infections

- Eye problems (including cataracts)
- Headache
- Muscle weakness
- Unusual increase in facial hair growth
- Menstruation problems
- Thinning skin

BRMs

- Irritation at site of injection
- Nausea or upset stomach
- Headache
- Cold symptoms
- Abdominal pain
- Unusual tiredness
- Fever
- Vomiting
- Rash and itching

OTHER PRECAUTIONS

NSAIDs

- These medications can make you drowsy. Make sure you know how they affect you before you do anything that requires your full alertness.
- These medications have been known to affect pregnancies and can pass into breast milk. Some studies show that this type of medication interferes with the production of the fatty acids needed to implant an embryo in the womb and are associated with an increase in the risk of miscarriage. Check with your doctor if you are pregnant or nursing.
- NSAIDs should not be taken if you are allergic to aspirin. The combination can cause serious side effects. Ibuprofen and naproxen also should not be taken if you are having any kind of surgery as they can increase your chances of bleeding during the surgery.

- If you are allergic to aspirin, check the label of any other anti-inflammatory very carefully. Many of them have aspirin as a major ingredient.

- Do not combine aspirin and other NSAIDs or you may be double dosing on aspirin.

- These medications also should not be taken if you are having any kind of surgery as they can increase your chances of bleeding during the surgery.

COX-2 Inhibitors

- Alcohol and COX-2 inhibitors may increase your risk for gastrointestinal (GI) problems.

- These medications have been known to affect pregnancies and can pass into breast milk. Check with your doctor if you are pregnant or nursing.

OTC Analgesics

- Acetaminophen may cause liver damage when used with alcohol. It is a good idea to avoid alcohol if you are on any of this medication. This medication should be used with caution if you have a history of ANY alcohol abuse

- Acetaminophen should not be used in patients with G6PD (Glucose-6-phosphate dehydrogenase) deficiency, a metabolic disorder than can lead to anemia.

- Overdose of acetaminophen is very difficult to treat. The maximum dose equals two 500mg tablets (extra-strength Tylenol) four times a day.

Prescription Analgesics

- Some prescription analgesics are narcotics and they will add to the effects of alcohol.

- Narcotic analgesics can become habit forming. Although Tramadol is not a narcotic, it can also become habit forming. Check the list of symptoms of dependency on page 9 and contact your doctor if you are experiencing these symptoms.

◎ These medications have been known to affect pregnancies and can pass into breast milk. Check with your doctor if you are pregnant or nursing.

DMARDs

◎ DMARDs can affect a pregnancy through the mother or the father.

◎ Some DMARDs should absolutely not be used if you are pregnant as they can cause abortion. Check this carefully with your doctor.

◎ These medications may pass into breast milk. You may want to consider bottle-feeding if you are taking this type of medication.

◎ DMARDs may take a few months to begin working so you will probably need to take other medications also.

◎ These medications suppress your immune system so check with your doctor before taking any vaccinations for other diseases.

◎ Drinking alcohol while on these medications can increase the chance of liver problems.

◎ Grapefruit juice can interfere with the effectiveness of these medications.

◎ Sulfasalazine is a sulfa drug and should not be taken if you are allergic to sulfa drugs.

◎ Sulfasalazine can make your skin more sensitive to the sun. Make sure you take proper precautions when in the sun and avoid tanning booths and sun lamps.

◎ Sulfasalazine can affect sperm count and sperm function.

◎ Sulfasalazine can turn your urine an orange-yellow color and may also stain contact lenses.

Immunosuppressants

◎ Drinking alcohol can increase the side effects of these medications. Be sure to check that other medications you might be taking, like cough syrups, do not contain alcohol.

◎ These medications suppress your immune system and may interfere with your body's ability to fight other infections while you are on it. Long-term use could lead to lymphoma and liver problems.

◎ These medications have been known to affect pregnancies and can pass into breast milk. Check with your doctor if you are pregnant or nursing.

◎ These medications can reduce sperm count and there is a higher incidence of miscarriages if the male's partner does conceive.

Corticosteroids

◎ Corticosteroids should not be stopped without supervision from your doctor. Abruptly stopping this type of medication can have serious side effects.

◎ Because long-term use of corticosteroids lowers your resistance to infections, check with your doctor before having a vaccination or before making plans to be with others who have been vaccinated.

◎ Oral contraceptives may also increase the side effects of corticosteroids.

◎ These medications have been known to affect pregnancies and can pass into breast milk. Check with your doctor if you are pregnant or nursing.

BRMs

◎ BRMs are relatively new drugs and there is little information about long-term risks. Their safety during pregnancy or nursing is not known. Check with your doctor about the possible risks.

◎ These medications suppress your immune system and may interfere with your body's ability to fight other infections while you are on them.

THE BOTTOM LINE

There are many other prescription and nonprescription medications for JRA that are not mentioned. Your doctor will let you know which is the right one for you. You can get a general idea of how the medication works and what the side effects are if you know what type of medication it is.

Some of the drugs work better when combined and some have more dangerous side effects when combined. Check with your doctor and follow the instructions carefully before taking these medications in combination.

As with any medications, you may experience side effects that are not on the list. If you experience anything out of the ordinary, contact your doctor right away. Other side effects are less common, but they may affect you.

While the list of side effects appears daunting, it is very important that you take the medication as prescribed. Inform you doctor of any unusual side effects, either listed or not. It is possible that the medication can be adjusted to minimize those effects.

It is important to exercise when your symptoms allow it. Exercise keeps your joints mobile and keeps your muscles strong. If you are experiencing a flare-up of your symptoms, you can limit your exercise, but you should continue, under the supervision of your doctor, when you are able. Swimming is a good exercise because it uses many of your joints and muscles without putting weight on your joints.

There is a lot of research going on in the area of JRA. Scientists are studying the causes of the disease and are successfully developing new drugs to reduce inflammation and to slow the progression of the disease. Don't give up hope.

You may need to have your school program modified when you are having a flare-up of your symptoms or to accommodate the side effects of the medications you are taking. This is not a crutch. It is what you need to be successful in school and you may be eligible for a Special Education plan or a 504-accommodation plan. Some possible accommodations are:

- Late arrival at school if it is difficult for you to get started in the morning due to stiffness or drowsiness as a side effect of the medication.
- A separate place to work if you are taking medications that increase your susceptibility to infection.
- Modified requirements in physical education classes until your medication starts to work.

13 Kidney Disease

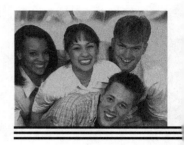

The kidney diseases addressed in this chapter are nephritis, an inflammation or infection in the filtering units of your kidneys, and nephrosis, damage to the filtering units. Both of these conditions cause your kidneys to lose proteins and red blood cells through your urine because of the inflammation or damage to the filtering system. As the amount of protein in the blood decreases, fluid builds up and parts of your body, such as around your hands, feet, and eyes, swell up. Without proper treatment, this damage can cause the kidneys to stop working properly.

THE MOST COMMON PRESCRIPTION MEDICATIONS

Corticosteroid Anti-Inflammatory Drugs

Prednisone (Deltasone®)

Diuretics

Loop Diuretics

Furosemide (Lasix®)

Bumetanide (Bumex®)

Torsemide (Demadex®)

Ethacryinic acid (Edecrin®)

Thiazide Diuretics

Hydrochlorothiazide (Esidrix)

Chlorothiazide (Diuril®)

Methyclothiazide (Enduron®)

Bendroflumethiazide (Naturetin®)

Potassium-Sparing Diuretics

Amiloride (Midamor®)

Triamterene (Dyrenium®)

Spironolactone (Aldactone®)

GENERAL INFORMATION ABOUT HOW THESE DRUGS WORK

Kidney diseases can result from different reasons. Medications are prescribed to curb the inflammation in the filtering units, to treat the underlying cause of the problem if it is known, and to ease the symptoms of the disease, such as anemia and fluid retention.

Corticosteroid anti-inflammatory drugs block the release of chemicals in the body that produce inflammation and suppress the activity of your immune system. They affect the body's ability to maintain inflammation.

Diuretics increase the rate of urine flow because they increase the rate at which the sodium is eliminated from your body. They decrease blood pressure because they decrease the amount of fluid in the cells and allow for easier blood flow. The different diuretics accomplish this by working on the kidneys in different ways. Loop diuretics block the absorption of salt and fluid from the kidney tubules and increase urine output. They also inhibit the "pump" that cycles the sodium back into the bloodstream. Thiazide diuretics block the movement of sodium and fluids in the kidneys and this increases urine production. They inhibit sodium reabsorption and therefore increase urinary excretion of water and sodium.

Potassium-sparing diuretics interfere with the level of sodium and fluid retention in the kidneys but they block the excretion of potassium when sodium is excreted. Amiloride and Triamterene block a sodium channel and interfere with the passage of sodium and increase the urinary excretion of sodium. Spironolactone interferes with the binding of the hormone aldosterone, a hormone in your body that causes sodium and water retention. This retention is in response to your body's secreting too much potassium.

THE MOST COMMON POSSIBLE SIDE EFFECTS

Corticosteroids

- Short term:
  - Fluid retention and weight gain
  - Slow healing of wounds
  - Easy bruising
  - Increased appetite
  - Indigestion
  - Insomnia
- Long term:
  - Slow growth
  - Lowered resistance to infections
  - Eye problems (including cataracts)
  - Headache
  - Muscle weakness
  - Unusual increase in facial hair growth
  - Menstruation problems
  - Thinning skin

Loop Diuretics

- Dry mouth
- Increased thirst
- Unusual tiredness
- Weakness
- Muscle cramps

- Muscle pain
- Dizziness
- Lightheadedness
- Skin rash
- Abnormal heart rate

Thiazide Diuretics

- Dry mouth
- Increased thirst
- Weakness
- Muscle cramps or pain
- Low blood pressure
- Abnormal heart rate

Potassium-Sparing Diuretics—Spironolactone Only

- Breast enlargement in men
- Menstrual irregularities in women

OTHER PRECAUTIONS

Corticosteroids

- Corticosteroids should not be stopped without supervision from your doctor. Abruptly stopping this type of medication can have serious side effects.
- Because long-term use of corticosteroids lowers your resistance to infections, check with your doctor before having vaccinations or before making plans to be with others who have been vaccinated.
- Oral contraceptives may also increase the side effects of corticosteroids.
- These medications have been known to affect pregnancies and can pass into breast milk. Check with your doctor if you are pregnant or nursing.

Diuretics

◎ These medications have been known to affect pregnancies and can pass into breast milk. Check with your doctor if you are pregnant or nursing.

◎ Except for potassium-sparing diuretics, these medications rob your body of potassium. Many of the side effects associated with the medications are related to the loss of potassium and other electrolytes.

◎ These medications can make you drowsy. Make sure you know how they affect you before you do anything that requires your full alertness.

◎ These medications decrease blood pressure, so be careful when standing up quickly from a resting position.

◎ Drinking alcohol can make you feel dizzy or lightheaded while on this type of medication.

◎ Some of these medications are similar in structure to sulfa, so you should not take those if you are allergic to sulfa. Check this out carefully with your doctor.

◎ Nonsteroidal anti-inflammatory drugs (NSAIDs) have caused elevated potassium levels and they may blunt the diuretic effects of these drugs and should not be used if you have kidney disease.

◎ Spironolactone is similar in structure to steroids and may have sexual side effects such as impotence in men and bleeding irregularities in women.

THE BOTTOM LINE

Kidney disease is usually caused by some other medical condition, such as high blood pressure, diabetes, lupus, infections, and inflammation. Therefore, you are probably taking medications for those problems as well. Make sure you let your kidney specialist know of any other medications or alternative remedies you are taking. Since many prescription and over-the-counter medications are cleared from your body through your kidneys, make sure you tell your doctor and pharmacists about any medications or alternative remedies you are taking to make sure they don't make your condition worse.

In kidney disease there is a decrease in your production of erythropoietin (EPO)—a hormone that enables your body to make red blood cells. Your body needs red blood cells to carry oxygen where it is needed. You may need to take epoetin alfa (Procrit®), a man-made form of the hormone. It is given by injection and can cause joint pain, irritation at the injection site, headache, fatigue, vomiting, and diarrhea.

Diet and lifestyle changes are important as well as taking the medication. You will not always be able to eat the same foods or stay up as late as your friends. You may need to control the amount of protein, sodium, and phosphorus you eat. Alcohol can be a greater risk for you than it is for your friends. Make sure you have a medical person you feel comfortable with who can help you with all of the things you need to know and the precautions you need to take. You might also work with a dietician to make sure you keep a healthy diet that is right for you.

You may need to take many different medications and supplements in order to manage your disease and it could be difficult to keep track of it all. An alarm clock or watch can let you know when it is time to take your medications.

Some of the side effects of the medications you need to take can be especially disturbing at this time. Long-term use of corticosteroids can cause weight gain and acne, problems you don't need at this time in your life. However, the side effects of not treating the condition can be worse. A support group or therapist can help you deal with these issues.

If medication and lifestyle changes don't work, it is possible you will need to start a procedure called dialysis. This is an artificial filtering system that does the filtering job that the kidneys can no longer do. If you need dialysis on a permanent basis, you will probably need a new kidney or kidney transplant.

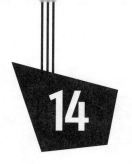

14

Lupus (Systemic Lupus Erythematosus—SLE)

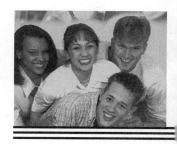

Lupus is a disorder of the immune system. Your body attacks your healthy cells and tissues leading to inflammation and damage to many parts of your body including your joints, skin, kidneys, heart, lungs, blood systems, and brain.

THE MOST COMMON MEDICATIONS

Anti-Inflammatory Drugs

Over-the-Counter Nonsteroidal Anti-Inflammatory Drugs (NSAIDs)

Ibuprofen (Advil®)

Ketoprofen (Orudis®)

Naproxen (Aleve®)

Prescription Nonsteroidal Anti-Inflammatory Drugs (NSAIDs)

Sulindac (Clinoril®)

Diclofenac (Voltaren®)

Piroxicam (Feldene®)

Diflunisal (Dolobid®)

Meloxicam (Mobic®)

Nabumetone (Relafen®)

Etodolac (Lodine®)

Oxaprozin (Daypro®)

Indomethacin (Indocin®)

Prescription COX-2 Inhibitors

Celecoxib (Celebrex®)

Prescription Corticosteroids

Prednisone (Deltasone®)

Methylprednisolone (Medrol®)

Dexamethasone (Decadron®)

Prescription Corticosteroid Creams

Clobetasol (Temovate®)

Halobetasol (Ultravate®)

Hydrocortisone (Dermacort®)

Triamcinolone (Aristocort®)

Betamethasone (Diprolene®)

Fluocinolone (Synalar®)

Fluocinonide (Lidex®)

Prescription Antimalarials

Hydroxychloroquine (Plaquenil®)

Chloroquine (Aralen®)

Prescription Immunosuppressants

Azathioprine (Imuran®)

Cyclophosphamide (Cytoxan®)

Methotrexate (Rheumatrex®)

Cyclosporine (Sandimmune®)

GENERAL INFORMATION ABOUT HOW THESE DRUGS WORK

The cause of lupus is unknown and currently there is no cure. The medications are designed to alleviate symptoms that generally include extreme fatigue, painful or swollen joints, unexplained fever, skin rashes, and kidney problems. They also work to minimize damage to your other organs.

NSAIDs work by blocking your body's production of specific hormones and chemicals that contribute to inflammation and pain. The OTC medications control pain. The prescriptive dose also controls the underlying inflammation. Some NSAIDs block one hormone and others block more than one.

The COX-2 inhibitors are NSAIDs that do not block the hormone that helps maintain the protective lining in your stomach.

Corticosteroids can ease the inflammation to the joints and organs. They block the release of chemicals in the body that produce inflammation and suppress the activity of your immune system.

Corticosteroid creams also appear to block the formation of chemicals in the body that produce inflammation and that cause swelling, redness, itching, and pain.

It is not quite clear how antimalarials work on lupus, but scientists think these medications suppress certain chemicals that cause inflammation. This has an anti-inflammatory effect and may prevent flare-ups from recurring.

Immunosuppressants target cells that grow at a fast rate and are able to block the action of some immune cells and interfere with the action of other immune cells that cause inflammation. These may be taken orally or intravenously.

THE MOST COMMON POSSIBLE SIDE EFFECTS

NSAIDs

- Diarrhea
- Nausea
- Vomiting
- Stomach cramps and pain
- Gas

COX-2 Inhibitors

- Headache
- Heartburn

- Gas
- Nausea
- Acid or sour stomach
- Abdominal pain
- Diarrhea
- Respiratory infection

Corticosteroids

- Short term:
  - Fluid retention and weight gain
  - Slow healing of wounds
  - Easy bruising
  - Increased appetite
  - Indigestion
  - Insomnia
- Long term:
  - Slow growth
  - Lowered resistance to infections
  - Eye problems (including cataracts)
  - Headache
  - Muscle weakness
  - Unusual increase in facial hair growth
  - Menstruation problems
  - Thinning skin

Corticosteroid Creams

- Burning
- Itching
- Irritation
- Acne
- Dry and cracking skin

Antimalarials (Few Common Side Effects but the Possibility of the Following)

- Diarrhea
- Vision problems
- Headache
- Itching
- Loss of appetite
- Nausea or vomiting
- Stomach cramps or pain

Immunosuppressants

- Nausea or vomiting
- Loss of appetite
- Darkening of the skin or fingernails
- Hair loss or increased hair growth on body and face
- Sterility in men (usually temporary)
- Reduced ability to fight infections
- Swollen or bleeding gums
- High blood pressure
- Hand tremors
- Kidney problems

OTHER PRECAUTIONS

NSAIDs

- These medications can make you drowsy. Make sure you know how they affect you before you do anything that requires your full alertness.

- These medications have been known to affect pregnancies and can pass into breast milk. Some studies show that this type of medication interferes with the production of the fatty acids needed to implant an embryo in the womb and are associated with an increase in the risk of miscarriage. Check with your doctor if you are pregnant or nursing.

- NSAIDs should not be taken if you are allergic to aspirin. The combination can cause serious side effects. Ibuprofen and naproxen also should not be taken if you are having any kind of surgery as they can increase your chances of bleeding during the surgery.
- Many nonsteroidal anti-inflammatory drugs are listed above. It is possible that one will work better for you than others. Also one may work for a while and then stop working as well. You may need to change to a different one to get the desired effects. Don't get discouraged if that happens. There are many choices so talk with your doctor about what to try next.

COX-2 Inhibitors

- Alcohol and COX-2 inhibitors may increase your risk for gastrointestinal (GI) problems.
- These medications have been known to affect pregnancies and can pass into breast milk. Check with your doctor if you are pregnant or nursing.

Corticosteroids

- Corticosteroids should not be stopped without supervision from your doctor. Abruptly stopping this type of medication can have serious side effects.
- Because long-term use of corticosteroids lowers your resistance to infections, check with your doctor before having a vaccination or before making plans to be with others who have been vaccinated.
- Oral contraceptives may also increase the side effects of corticosteroids.
- These medications have been known to affect pregnancies and can pass into breast milk. Check with your doctor if you are pregnant or nursing.

Antimalarials

- These medications have been known to affect pregnancies and can pass into breast milk. Check with your doctor if you are pregnant or nursing.

- There are vision problems associated with this type of medication. Do not drive or engage in other activities that require precise vision until you know how this medication will affect you.

Immunosuppressants

- Immunosuppressants can affect the cells that are causing your problems as well as healthy cells. Many of the side effects are due to their affect on your healthy cells.

- These medications suppress your immune system so check with your doctor before taking any vaccinations for other diseases.

- These medications have been known to affect pregnancies (through the mother and the father) and can pass into breast milk. Check with your doctor if you are pregnant or nursing.

- Grapefruit juice can interfere with the effectiveness of some of these medications.

THE BOTTOM LINE

It is important to receive regular care with lupus rather than just during a flare-up.

There is much research going on looking for more effective treatments and a cure for lupus. Your doctor may prescribe a medication that is not on this list. Be sure to ask the same questions about that medication to make sure you stay informed and an integral part of your treatment.

You may be seeing many different specialists due to how your lupus affects your body. Be sure you let them know about each other and the medications prescribed by each one. Make sure you have a comfortable working relationship with all of your health care providers.

There may be other drugs you need to take that deal with complications of your disease, such as fluid retention, seizures, or high blood pressure. Make sure you let your doctor know all medications and any alternative remedies you are taking to make sure there are no adverse interactions between them.

There may be additional side effects from these medications if you have other medical conditions. Make sure your doctor knows any other conditions that you have or have had in the past.

Smoking, drinking, and taking drugs can have a bad interaction with the medications you are taking. Check with your doctor about any possible interactions.

Because of the increased risk of infections from many of the medications, tattooing and body piercing are especially forbidden.

If you are having difficulty taking your medications because of the stomach upset they cause, talk with your doctor or pharmacist. It is possible that they can be taken in different ways or in different dosages to minimize that problem.

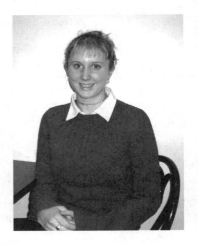

I was diagnosed with lyme disease when I was 16 years old. I saw a variety of doctors and had many tests before the conclusion was made. At first the doctor thought I was making up the symptoms and I was treated for a virus and was put on Amoxycylin®. It kept the symptoms in check but it didn't get rid of the disease. I was tested for a brain tumor and a stroke because I was partially paralyzed on one side, had memory loss, and my left hand seized into a claw position. Tests for lyme disease came back borderline negative so the doctor ruled that out. I finally found a doctor who specializes in infectious diseases and he made the diagnosis right away. He said that it is common for the test to come back borderline negative and began treating me for lyme disease. It took one and a half years of medications before I was functional and I lost a year of school. The medications made me worse for about two weeks and I was worried they weren't going to work. The fatigue was worse and all of the symptoms were exaggerated. Since then it has been a slow but steady upward trend. Currently, I am taking Plaquenil® and Biaxin®. The medicines I take change about every three-month cycles because my body builds up a resistance. The other medications that I changed to are Tetracycline® and Minocycline®. When I change the combinations, there is a one and a half- to two-week slump while adjusting to the new meds. The doctor prescribed pain medications for the aches and pains, but I didn't like the "out of it" feeling, so I don't take it.

I try not to take the medications at school because it is difficult to get to the nurse's office at the right time. Luckily my meds aren't so strict about when they need to be taken just as long as there is a significant period of time between the two doses. I can take them at home so I don't have to take them at school. The Tetracycline® caused acne and severe sunburn. I was sitting in a car and got a burn on the arm near the window. I couldn't go outside without being totally covered when I was on it. The Plaquenil® can cause vision problems, so I see an eye doctor every three months. So far there are no problems. The Biaxin® ruins whatever you are eating. The Minocycline® caused dizziness and fainting spells. I got a concussion once when I fell down the stairs due to a fainting spell. I didn't care for the Minocycline®.

My doctor wants to take me off all medication soon because I have been doing so well lately, but I'm sending out college applications and the last thing I want is to get really sick. So I will stay on them until that is over. I went off the meds one and a half years into the illness when I was showing progress. My memory loss came back and I was sleeping fifteen to twenty hours daily.

I work closely with my new primary care doctor and the infectious disease doctor. I use a day planner for my appointments and put down when the medications are changed and list all the symptoms on the side. I have a special day planner just for medical issues. If there are any changes in the symptoms, I let the doctor know. The infectious diseases doctor is out of the country a lot, so we often communicate by e-mail.

The major problem I hear in my support group is that people will only stick with a medication for one month because they don't see results and then they try something else. My advice is to stick with it because it is a very long and slow process. I am glad I stuck with it. My focus now is how I can maintain a normal life and normal schedule.
— Allison, age 19, senior in high school, lyme disease (The antimalarial drug she takes for her lyme disease is also prescribed for lupus.)

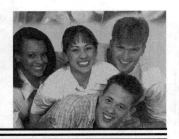

Migraines

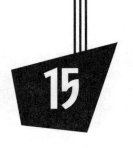

Migraines are debilitating, throbbing headaches that usually occur on one side of the head. They are usually accompanied by nausea, vomiting, and sensitivity to light and sound.

THE MOST COMMON MEDICATIONS

Pain Relievers

Over-the-Counter Analgesic Medications

Acetaminophen (Tylenol®)

Aspirin (Arthritis Pain Formula®)

Aspirin/Acetaminophen/Caffeine (Excedrin Migraine®)

Prescription Narcotic and Sedative Analgesics

Propoxyphene/Aspirin/Caffeine (Darvon Compound®)

Propoxyphene/Acetaminophen (Darvocet-N®)

Oxycodone/Aspirin (Percodan®)

Oxycodone/Acetaminophen (Percocet®)

Aspirin/Codeine (Empirin with codeine®)

Acetaminophen/Codeine (Tylenol with Codeine®)

Aspirin/Butalbital/Caffeine (Fiorinal®)

Acetaminophen/Butalbital (Phrenilin®)

Acetaminophen/Butalbital/Caffeine (Esgic®)

Isometheptene/Acetaminophen/Dichloralphenazone (Midrin®)

Over-the-Counter Nonsteroidal Anti-Inflammatory Drugs (NSAIDs)

Ibuprofen (Advil®)

Naproxen (Aleve®)

Ketoprofen (Orudis®)

Prescription Antinausea Medications

Prochlorperazine (Compazine®)

Promethazine (Phenergan®)

Metoclopramide (Reglan®)

Prescription Attack Stoppers

Ergot Alkaloids

Ergotamine (Ergostat®)

Ergotamine/Caffeine (Wigraine®)

Dihydroergotamine (DHE-45®—injectable)

Dihydroergotamine (Migranal®—nasal)

Triptans

Almotriptan (Axert®)

Frovatriptan (Frova®)

Naratriptan (Amerge®)

Rizatriptan (Maxalt®)

Sumatriptan (Imitrex®)

Zolmitriptan (Zomig®)

Prescription Attack Preventers

Tricyclic Antidepressants (TCAs)

Amitriptyline (Elavil®)

Nortriptyline (Pamelor®)

Doxepin (Sinequan®)

Protriptyline (Vivactil®)

Selective Serotonin Reuptake Inhibitors (SSRIs)

Fluoxetine (Prozac®)

Paroxetine (Paxil®)

Sertraline (Zoloft®)

Beta-Blockers

Propranolol (Inderal®)

Metoprolol (Lopressor®)

Timolol (Blocadren®)

Nadolol (Corgard®)

Atenolol (Tenormin®)

Calcium Channel Blockers

Verapamil (Isoptin®)

Diltiazem (Cardizem®)

Nifedipine (Adalat®)

Antihistamines

Cyproheptadine (Periactin®)

Anticonvulsants

Divalproex (Depakote®)

Gabapentin (Neurontin®)

Topiramate (Topamax®)

Neurotoxin

Botulinum Toxin (Botox®)

GENERAL INFORMATION ABOUT HOW THESE DRUGS WORK

The cause of migraines is not completely clear or the same with each person. One theory is that the headaches are a result of the narrowing and widening of the blood vessels in the brain and many of the medications are designed to treat that occurrence. There is also research to support that migraines are a result of a disorder of the central nervous system that includes the brain, the nerves, and the blood vessels. Other migraine medications act on the central nervous system.

Early Hungarians used a mixture of rosemary and sugar to treat headaches. Hawaiians applied ginger root juice and coarse salt to the head. The Egyptians made a compress from the oil of castor beans. Finns ate or applied horseradish to redirect blood flow. Dian Dincin Buchman, *Ancient Healing Secrets: Practical Cures That Work Today* (Baltimore: Ottenheimer, 1996).

The focus of migraine medications is to relieve the symptoms of a migraine headache so that you can function at or near normal levels and to decrease the frequency and severity of future attacks. Treatment is recommended to either to stop an attack when it occurs, to treat the symptoms of the attack, or to prevent attacks from occurring. If you have headaches often, you may need a preventive medication on a regular basis.

Over-the-counter analgesic medications are thought to control pain by lowering your pain threshold. They should be taken as soon as you feel the attack or sense that an attack is imminent (an aura) to try to stop it.

Prescription narcotic and sedative analgesics are a combination of an analgesic or aspirin, which lowers your pain threshold with a narcotic or sedative. These combinations can provide better relief from pain than either one can do alone. The narcotics act on the central nervous system. Sedatives induce sleep and sleep can help relieve a migraine. Caffeine is added because it enhances the pain-relieving effect of aspirin or acetaminophen. With Midrin®, isometheptene narrows the blood vessels, acetaminophen lowers the pain threshold, and dichloralphenazone provides a sedative effect.

NSAIDs work by blocking your body's production of specific hormones and chemicals that contribute to inflammation and pain.

Some antinausea medications are thought to prevent the nausea that often accompanies migraines by affecting the dopamine receptors in your brain. This helps because dopamine can cause nausea. They also are thought to secrete hormones that improve the absorption of other antimigraine medications you are taking because they speed up the emptying of your stomach. Others are thought to work on the part of the brain that controls vomiting, but the way they work is unclear.

Ergot alkaloids are vasoconstrictors that help counteract the painful dilation stage of the headache by constricting the dilated blood vessels or by helping reduce blood vessel inflammation. Combining ergot alkaloids with caffeine promotes absorption. These drugs will not prevent the headache.

Triptans are developed specifically to fight migraines. They affect a specific serotonin receptor and narrow the blood vessels in your brain that become widened during an attack. They can alleviate many of the symptoms as well as the pain but cannot prevent an attack. They should be taken at the very first sign of an attack.

Tricyclic antidepressants affect the transmission of the neurotransmitters norepinephrine and serotonin. They block the passage of these chemicals as they go in and out of the nerve endings and raise the levels of them in the brain. This produces a sedative effect.

Some studies have shown that certain serotonin levels decrease, causing blood vessels to dilate as migraine symptoms get worse. SSRIs block the neurotransmitter serotonin from moving into the nerve endings. Therefore, more is available surrounding the nerve endings and its action is increased.

Beta-blockers interfere with the action of the part of the nervous system that controls the pace of your heart. They can reduce the frequency of migraines by reducing blood vessel constriction.

Getting a head start on migraine pain

Research shows why it's important for migraine sufferers to take prescription drugs called triptans promptly.

1. The pain of migraine begins when peripheral nerves near blood vessels get irritated and hyper-excited.

2. Signals from the blood vessels are transmitted via a network of peripheral neurons in the spinal cord.

3. Neurons in the spinal cord and thalamus relay signals from peripheral neurons to the upper brain, where pain is perceived. The nerve from the eye sockets relays sensory signals to central neurons in the spinal cord. The brain can misinterpret the eye sockets as the source of the pain.

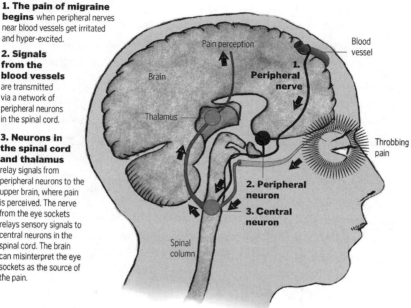

Pain perception

Blood vessel

Brain

1. Peripheral nerve

Thalamus

Throbbing pain

2. Peripheral neuron

3. Central neuron

Spinal column

What the medication does

Triptans calm the peripheral nerves and block communication with central neurons. The drugs have no effect on central neurons.

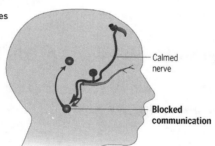

Calmed nerve

Blocked communication

Time sensitive
In most people who get migraines, the central neurons also become sensitized and begin firing on their own accord, usually an hour or two after the onset of pain.

Too late
The sensitized central neurons continue to send pain signals, even if peripheral neurons are calmed.

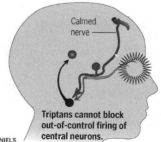

Calmed nerve

Triptans cannot block out-of-control firing of central neurons.

SOURCES: Rami Burstein, Moshe Jakubowski; graphic based on drawings by Jakubowski

GLOBE STAFF GRAPHIC/DAVID BUTLER, CINDY DANIELS

How Migraine Medication Works
Rami Burstein and Moshe Jakubowski, "Stopping Migraine Pain," *The Boston Globe*, **6 January 2004, p. C1.**

Calcium channel blockers affect the passage of calcium into the muscle cells in your blood vessels and cause the blood vessels to relax. This lowers blood pressure.

Antihistamines block the action of histamines that are released when your body encounters an allergen and the antihistamine dries up secretions in your nose, throat, and eyes. In migraines, the sedative effect helps decrease the vomiting associated with the migraines. Cyproheptadine is also thought to interfere with the movement of serotonin in the brain.

Anticonvulsants are thought to improve the activity of GABA (gamma-amniobutynic acid), the major inhibitor of nerve transmission in the brain, by increasing the amount of GABA in the brain. The increased amount of neurotransmitter available may have a stabilizing effect on the cells in your brain. The exact way they work with migraines is not fully known.

Doctors are not quite sure how Botox works with migraines. They think it blocks the sensory nerves that carry pain messages to the brain and cause muscles to relax so there is less sensitivity to the pain.

THE MOST COMMON POSSIBLE SIDE EFFECTS

Over-the-Counter Analgesic Medications Containing Aspirin

- Nausea
- Upset stomach or cramps
- Heartburn
- Gastrointestinal bleeding
- Vomiting

Prescription Narcotic and Sedative Analgesics

- Lightheadedness
- Drowsiness
- Nausea
- Vomiting

◎ Upset stomach or pain

◎ Shortness of breath

◎ Constipation

◎ Dizziness

NSAIDs

◎ Diarrhea

◎ Nausea

◎ Vomiting

◎ Stomach cramps or pain

◎ Gas

Antinausea Medications

Metoclopramide

◎ Restlessness

◎ Drowsiness

◎ Depression

◎ Rash and itching

◎ Sleeplessness

Prochlorperazine and Promethazine

◎ Reduced sweating

◎ Dry mouth

◎ Blurred vision

◎ Drowsiness

◎ Uncontrolled movements after long-term use

◎ Stiffness and walking difficulties after long-term use

Ergot Alkaloids

◎ Dizziness

◎ Drowsiness

◎ Nausea

- Vomiting
- Diarrhea
- Cold and tingling in hands and feet

Triptans

- Increase in blood pressure
- Heaviness and tightness in the chest
- Nausea
- Drowsiness
- Tingling in hands and feet
- Dry mouth
- Headache
- Dizziness
- Hot flashes
- Vomiting
- Irritation and pain at site of injection
- Weakness
- Lightheadedness
- Muscle aches or stiffness
- Sweating

TCAs

- Blurred vision
- Dry mouth
- Dizziness or lightheadedness
- Constipation
- Difficulty urinating
- Sensitivity to bright light
- Weight changes
- Drowsiness
- Headache
- Increased appetite
- Nausea
- Unpleasant taste in the mouth

SSRIs

- Headache
- Anxiety
- Nervousness
- Sleeplessness
- Drowsiness
- Tiredness
- Weakness
- Changes in sex drive
- Tremors
- Sweating
- Appetite loss
- Nausea
- Diarrhea
- Skin rash
- Itching

Beta-Blockers

- Sexual difficulties
- Dizziness or lightheadedness
- Drowsiness
- Sleeplessness
- Unusual tiredness or weakness

Calcium Channel Blockers

- Swelling of feet and legs
- Dizziness
- Constipation
- Weakness
- Headache
- Flushing or feeling of warmth
- Nausea

Antihistamines

◎ Dry mouth or nose

◎ Drowsiness

Anticonvulsants

◎ Nausea

◎ Vomiting

◎ Indigestion

◎ Sedation

◎ Unusual weight changes

◎ Loss of appetite

◎ Tremors

◎ Diarrhea

◎ Hair loss

◎ Dizziness

◎ Unusual tiredness or weakness

◎ Abnormal eye movements or twitching or blurred or double vision

◎ Clumsiness or unsteadiness

◎ Slow reflexes

◎ Difficulty concentrating

◎ Memory problems

◎ Speech and language problems

Neurotoxin

◎ Weakness in the muscle where it was injected

◎ Injection site reactions such as pain and bleeding

OTHER PRECAUTIONS

Over-the-Counter Analgesic Medications

◎ If you are taking over-the-counter medications like Excedrin Migraine, don't take longer than ten consecutive days.

- Acetaminophen may cause liver damage when used with alcohol. It is a good idea to avoid alcohol if you are on this medication. This medication should be used with caution if you have a history of ANY alcohol abuse.

- Acetaminophen should not be used in patients with G6PD (Glucose-6-phosphate dehydrogenase) deficiency, a metabolic disorder than can lead to anemia.

- Overdose of acetaminophen is very difficult to treat. The maximum dose equals two 500mg tablets (Extra-strength Tylenol) four times a day.

- If you are allergic to aspirin, check the label of any other anti-inflammatory or pain medication very carefully. Many of them have aspirin as a major ingredient.

- Medications containing aspirin should not be taken if you are having any kind of surgery as they can increase your chances of bleeding during the surgery.

- Do not combine aspirin and other NSAIDs or you may be double dosing on aspirin.

Prescription Narcotic and Sedative Analgesics

- Narcotics can interfere with brain function and can be addictive when used for long periods of time. Take these carefully under the supervision of your doctor.

- Some prescriptive analgesics are narcotics and they will add to the effects of alcohol.

- These medications have been known to affect pregnancies and can pass into breast milk. Check with your doctor if you are pregnant or nursing.

NSAIDs

- These medications can make you drowsy. Make sure you know how they affect you before you do anything that requires your full alertness.

- These medications have been known to affect pregnancies and can pass into breast milk. Some studies show that this type of medication interferes with the production of the fatty acids needed to implant an embryo in the womb and are associated with an increase in the risk of miscarriage. Check with your doctor if you are pregnant or nursing

◎ NSAIDs should not be taken if you are allergic to aspirin. The combination can cause serious side effects. Ibuprofen and naproxen also should not be taken if you are having any kind of surgery as they can increase your chances of bleeding during the surgery.

Antinausea Medications

◎ These medications can add to the effects of alcohol and other central nervous system depressants.

◎ These medications have been known to affect pregnancies and can pass into breast milk. Check with your doctor if you are pregnant or nursing.

Ergot Alkaloids

◎ These can increase the risk of abortion if used while you are pregnant.

◎ These medications may pass into breast milk. You may want to consider bottle-feeding if you are taking this type of medication.

◎ These medications restrict blood vessels in the brain but could also constrict them in other parts of the body resulting in a lack of sufficient blood supply to other organs.

◎ Alcohol can make your headaches worse, especially if you are taking ergotamines.

◎ These medications can make you drowsy. Make sure you know how they affect you before you do anything that requires your full alertness.

Triptans

◎ Oral contraceptives can interact with triptan-type drugs and increase the levels of these drugs in the blood thereby elevating the side effects.

◎ Triptan-type drugs are not recommended for people under the age of eighteen.

- These medications can make you drowsy. Make sure you know how they affect you before you do anything that requires your full alertness.
- These medications have been known to affect pregnancies and can pass into breast milk. Check with your doctor if you are pregnant or nursing.
- Do not take these medications while you are taking Monoamine Oxidase Inhibitors (MAOIs) because of an increased risk of side effects.

TCAs

- Smoking and oral contraceptives may reduce the effects of TCAs
- These medications can add to the effects of alcohol and other central nervous system depressants.
- These medications have been known to affect pregnancies and can pass into breast milk. Check with your doctor if you are pregnant or nursing.
- These medications can make your skin more sensitive to the sun. Make sure you take proper precautions when in the sun and avoid tanning booths and sun lamps.

SSRIs

- There has been a lot of controversy concerning prescribing these medications for patients under the age of eighteen. Work closely with your doctor if SSRIs have been prescribed for you.
- Do not stop taking antidepressants without talking with your doctor. Some of them have side effects that occur if you stop abruptly and you may need to taper off of the medication.
- These medications have been known to affect pregnancies and can pass into breast milk. Check with your doctor if you are pregnant or nursing.
- These medications can add to the effects of alcohol and other central nervous system depressants.
- These medications can make you drowsy. Make sure you know how they affect you before you do anything that requires your full alertness.

Beta-Blockers

⊚ Try to avoid competitive sports if you are on beta-blockers. These medications might interfere with your cardiac and cardiovascular response to the physical activity and may compromise your performance.

Calcium Channel Blockers

⊚ These medications have been known to affect pregnancies and can pass into breast milk. Check with your doctor if you are pregnant or nursing.

Antihistamine

⊚ These medications can add to the effects of alcohol and other central nervous system depressants.

Anticonvulsants

⊚ These medications can add to the effects of alcohol and other central nervous system depressants.

⊚ These medications have been known to affect pregnancies and can pass into breast milk. Check with your doctor if you are pregnant or nursing.

⊚ Oral contraceptives may be affected by these medications. The effectiveness of the oral contraceptives may be lowered.

Neurotoxin

⊚ Long-term effects of this treatment are not known.

⊚ It only affects the injected area and the effects wear off within a few months.

THE BOTTOM LINE

As you can see from the list, there are many different types of migraine medications. You will need to work closely with your doctor, and may need to try more than one type, to find what works for you. Some of the medications prescribed for migraines are typically used to treat other conditions. Usually the recommended dosages for migraines are different than those for the other disorders.

Medications for migraines are more effective when they are combined with lifestyle changes. Try to find out which activities and foods trigger migraines for you so that you can keep away from them. Exercise and relaxation and stress-reduction techniques have been know to help. It might be helpful to keep a headache diary of what triggered a migraine and what worked to get you out of it.

When headaches are so severe that these medications don't help, you might need to go to the hospital for stronger medications.

There has been a lot of publicity about whether Paxil or other SSRIs cause suicide. At this point, doctors don't know whether it is the result of the medications or the result of the condition, however it should make you more alert to questions about the medications you are using. A good working relationship with your doctor is especially important when you are on medications for migraines.

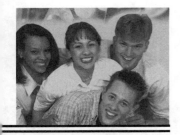

Seizure Disorders

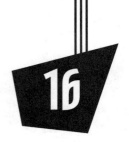

16

There are more than thirty different types of seizures. A seizure itself is a physical reaction to abnormal, excess discharges of the neurons in your brain. Epilepsy is an underlying disease of the brain that is manifest by recurring seizures.

THE MOST COMMON PRESCRIPTION MEDICATIONS

Anticonvulsants

Carbamazepine (Tegretol®)

Ethosuximide (Zarontin®)

Felbamate (Felbatol®)

Gabapentin (Neurontin®)

Lamotrigine (Lamictal®)

Levetiracetam (Keppra®)

Oxcarbazepine (Trileptal®)

Phenobarbital (Solfoton®)

Phenytoin (Dilantin®)

Primidone (Mysoline®)

Tiagabine (Gabatril®)

Topiramate (Topomax®)

Valproic acid (Depakene®)

Zonisamide (Zonegran®)

Benzodiazepines

Clonazepam (Klonopin®)

Lorazepam (Ativan®)

Diazepam (Valium®)

The ancient Greeks treated seizures with mistletoe, dog urine, purges and bloodletting. The ancient Romans treated them by banning certain foods, black clothing and bathing and prescribed drinking human blood. Medieval Christians believed that prayers could prevent seizures. King Charles II of England was treated with bloodletting, forced vomiting, laxatives and foot plasters made of pigeon dung. Dian Dincin Buchman, *Ancient Healing Secrets: Practical Cures That Work Today* (Baltimore: Ottenheimer, 1996).

GENERAL INFORMATION ABOUT HOW THESE DRUGS WORK

One half of the seizures that occur have no known cause. The others are linked to an injury to your brain, defects in the wiring of your brain, a chemical imbalance in your brain, or some combination of these factors. Most types of seizures can be controlled with medication. These medications do not cure a seizure disorder. They work to control the seizures and only work as long as you take them.

There are many different medications for seizures and many different types of seizures. Your doctor will make the determination as to which medications are right for your type of seizure disorder. Some of the medications are used alone and others are designed to be additional medications if the initial one does not control the seizures alone.

Anticonvulsants, in general, control nerve impulses in the brain. They act on the central nervous system to reduce the number and the severity of your seizures and to make it more difficult for seizures to start and continue. Different medications are prescribed for certain types of seizures because of the way they work. The exact ways these medications work is not fully known, but studies show that they appear to work in certain specific ways.

Carbamazepine is used for treating partial and generalized tonic-clonic (grand mal) seizures. It is thought to suppress the irregular and uncontrolled electrical activity in the nerve cells of your brain that can lead to seizures.

Ethosuximide is used to treat absence (petit mal) seizures. It is thought to slow the activity in certain parts of the brain and suppress the abnormal firing of neurons that causes the seizures.

Felbamate acts on the central nervous system and makes it more difficult for seizures to start or to continue by preventing the seizure impulse from spreading in the brain. The exact way it does this is not fully known. It is used to treat partial seizures.

Gabapentin, lamotrigine, oxcarbazepine, and tiagabine are thought to slow the activity in certain parts of the brain and suppress the abnormal firing of neurons that causes the seizures. They are used as add-on therapies to treat partial seizures and they can also be used alone.

Levetiracetam is used as an add-on to treat partial seizure disorders and can also be used alone. It is only used in combination with other anticonvulsants because it is not known to affect nerve transmissions. The exact way it works is not fully known.

Phenobarbital is used to treat both partial and generalized seizures. It is thought to act as a sedative and reduce the nerve impulses in the brain. It can be used in combination with other anticonvulsants.

Phenytoin is thought to slow the activity in certain parts of the brain and filter the firing of neurons that causes the seizures. It is used for treating partial and generalized tonic-clonic seizures.

Primidone is thought to slow the activity in certain parts of the brain and suppress the abnormal firing of neurons that causes the seizures. It is called a pro drug—it turns into phenobarbital once it is metabolized. It is used to treat tonic-clonic, partial, generalized, and myoclonic seizures (a brief, single or multiple, irregular muscle contraction that may or may not include a loss of consciousness).

Valproic acid is thought to slow the activity in certain parts of the brain and suppress the abnormal firing of neurons that causes the seizures. It is used to treat partial, generalized tonic-clonic, absence, and myoclonic seizures.

Topiramate is used along with other drugs to control partial seizures and generalized tonic-clonic seizures. Topiramate is thought to slow the activity in certain parts of the brain and suppress the abnormal firing of neurons that causes the seizures.

Zonisamide is used as an add-on therapy to treat partial seizures. It has also been used in other seizure types including generalized seizures, myoclonic seizures, and absence seizures. It is thought to affect the sodium and calcium flow in and out of the nerve cells.

Benzodiazepines are used to stop a seizure immediately. They are central nervous system depressants and act as a sedative or tranquilizer. They slow down your nervous system by helping the brain chemical gamma-aminobutyric acid (GABA) inhibit activity in some of the nerves in the brain.

THE MOST COMMON POSSIBLE SIDE EFFECTS

These medications affect the brain and central nervous system and are metabolized by the liver and the kidneys. Any changes in your body that are related to the brain, liver, and kidneys should be reported to your physician to determine if they are side effects of the medication you are taking.

The dosages for these medications need to be continually monitored to make sure a therapeutic level of medication is in your body at all times. As the dosage of the medication is increased, there is a greater chance for side effects.

Carbamazepine

- Dizziness
- Drowsiness
- Unsteadiness
- Nausea

- Vomiting
- Blurred vision

Ethosuximide

- Drowsiness
- Loss of appetite
- Nausea
- Vomiting
- Stomach cramps

Felbamate

- Sleepiness
- Headache
- Dizziness
- Nervousness
- Upset stomach
- Vomiting
- Constipation
- Nausea
- Loss of appetite
- Fever
- Black and blue marks on the skin

Gabapentin and Tiagabine

- Drowsiness
- Dizziness
- Unusual tiredness or weakness
- Abnormal eye movements or twitching

Lamotrigine

- Headache
- Dizziness

- Nausea
- Drowsiness
- Blurred or double vision
- Life-threatening skin rashes

Levetiracetam

- Tiredness
- Weakness
- Dizziness
- Increased susceptibility to infection
- Drowsiness

Oxcarbazepine

- Walking, balance, and coordination difficulties
- Dizziness
- Double vision
- Abdominal pain
- Nausea
- Vomiting
- Drowsiness

Phenobarbital

- Drowsiness
- Dizziness
- Hangover effect
- Clumsiness and unsteadiness
- Lightheadedness

Phenytoin

- Abnormal growth of the gums over the teeth
- Slurred speech at high doses

- Life-threatening skin rashes
- Mental confusion
- Uncontrolled eye movements
- Dizziness
- Nervousness
- Uncontrolled twitching
- Difficulty focusing
- Tiredness
- Irritability
- Trembling
- Drowsiness
- Numbness and tingling in hands and feet
- Facial hair growth in women
- Acne

Primidone

- Clumsiness
- Unsteadiness
- Impotence
- Dizziness

Topiramate

- Weight loss
- Diarrhea
- Nausea
- Slow reflexes
- Difficulty concentrating
- Memory problems
- Speech and language problems
- Drowsiness
- Dizziness
- Unusual tiredness or weakness
- Clumsiness or unsteadiness

- Tingling sensations
- Tremors
- Nausea
- Vision problems
- Nervousness

Valproic Acid

- Blood disorders
- Nausea
- Vomiting
- Indigestion
- Sedation
- Unusual weight changes
- Loss of appetite
- Tremors
- Diarrhea
- Hair loss

Zonisamide

- Sleepiness
- Loss of appetite
- Dizziness
- Headache
- Nausea
- Agitation and restlessness
- Irritability
- Drowsiness
- Sleeplessness

Benzodiazepines

- Drowsiness
- Unsteadiness

⊚ Dizziness

⊚ Lightheadedness

⊚ Slurred speech

OTHER PRECAUTIONS

Anticonvulsants

⊚ These medications can make you drowsy. Make sure you know how they affect you before you do anything that requires your full alertness.

⊚ Many of these medications can decrease the effectiveness of oral contraceptives. Discuss this with your doctor. You might want to use more than one type of contraceptive while you are on these medications.

⊚ These medications have been known to affect pregnancies and can pass into breast milk. Check with your doctor if you are pregnant or nursing.

⊚ Smoking can decrease the effectiveness of some of these medications.

⊚ As many of these medications can cause stomach upset, it is a good idea to take them at meal times if they upset your stomach and to drink lots of water throughout the day.

⊚ Some of the medications interfere with memory and concentration. You may need accommodations at school if you are on this type of medication.

⊚ These medications can add to the effects of alcohol and other central nervous system depressants.

⊚ For these medications to work effectively, there must be a relatively constant level of the medication in your body at all times. Therefore, the medications must be taken regularly without missing a dose.

⊚ Carbamazepine can have life-threatening blood reactions and fatal skin reactions.

⊚ Carbamazepine can make your skin more sensitive to the sun. Make sure you take proper precautions when in the sun and avoid tanning booths and sun lamps.

⊚ Felbamate may cause blood and liver problems.

- ◎ Lamotrigine may cause life-threatening rashes within the first two to eight weeks of treatment.
- ◎ Phenobarbital can be addictive if taken for an extended period of time.
- ◎ Oxcarbazepine may cause low blood sodium levels during the first three months of treatment.
- ◎ Valproic acid can cause severe liver disease that usually shows up within the first six months of treatment.
- ◎ Zonegram is a sulfa derivative so if you are allergic to sulfa, you should not take this drug.

Benzodiazepines

- ◎ Benzodiazepines are generally prescribed for short periods of time because you can develop a tolerance to them. That means that you may have to stop taking the medication or the dosage will have to be increased.
- ◎ These medications have been known to affect pregnancies and can pass into breast milk. Check with your doctor if you are pregnant or nursing.
- ◎ These medications can add to the effects of alcohol and other central nervous system depressants.

THE BOTTOM LINE

The number of possible side effects for these medications is high. You need to work closely with your doctor to discuss the pros and cons for taking medications for your seizure disorder and weigh the positives against the possible ill effects.

Do not switch medications without the advice of your doctor. They may appear to work in a similar manner and work for the same type of seizure, but they are not interchangeable. Also, check with your doctor before changing to a generic version, as the way they act in your body may be different because of how they are prepared.

It is a good idea to carry a medic alert card or wear a bracelet stating that you have a seizure disorder and are taking medications.

You might want to stop your medication if you have been seizure free for a reasonable period of time. Check this carefully with your doctor. If you stop your medication suddenly and unadvisedly, you may have more seizures that are harder to treat.

Seizure medications need to be decreased gradually. Do not stop taking any medication abruptly and without working closely with your physician. Seizures can result from abruptly stopping your medication and that type of seizure can be even more serious. Also take any medication exactly as directed. Do not vary from what you are told by your doctor or pharmacist.

If medication does not work, surgery may be recommended. Work very closely with your doctor to make sure you know all the risks and possible side effects of this type of action.

Sexually Transmitted Diseases (STDs)

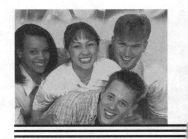

Sexually transmitted diseases are life-altering and life-threatening infections that you can get through sexual activity with someone who has that particular infection. The diseases include those caused by parasites: crabs (pubic lice), trichomoniasis, and scabies; those caused by viruses: hepatitis B and genital herpes, genital warts, human immunodeficiency virus/acquired immunodeficiency syndrome (HIV/AIDS); and those caused by bacteria: chlamydia, gonorrhea, and syphilis.

THE MOST COMMON PRESCRIPTION MEDICATIONS

Antiviral Drugs

Foscarnet (Foscavir®)

Ganciclovir (Cytovene®)

Acyclovir (Zovirax®)

Famciclovir (Famvir®)

Valacyclovir (Valtrex®)

Lamivudine (Eipivir®)

Adefovir (Hepsera®)

Biological Response Modifiers (BRMs)

Interferon-alpha (Intron A®)

Syphilis broke out in 1493 or 1494 during a dispute over the Kingdom of Naples. Spain and France were the major antagonists although the French soldiers, in particular, came from all over Europe. Initially, the disease was called the "disease of Naples," but it raged with such virulence among the French troops that France was forced to give up the campaign. When the army broke up and Polish, English, Hungarian, Swiss and German as well as French soldiers returned to their homes, the disease quickly became known as the "French Pox"—to everyone but the French.

Roy Porter, ed., *The Cambridge Illustrated History of Medicine* (Cambridge: Cambridge University Press, 1966).

Nucleoside Analogue Reverse Transcriptase Inhibitors (NRTIs)

Zidovudine-AZT (Retrovir®)

Didanosine (Videx®)

Zalcitabine (Hivid®)

Stavudine (Zerit®)

Abacavir (Ziagen®)

Protease Inhibitors (PIs)

Saquinavir (Fortovase®)

Ritonavir (Norvir®)

Indinavir (Crixivan®)

Nelfinavir (Viracept®)

Amprenavir (Agenerase®)

Lopinavir/Ritonavir (Kaletra®)

Nonnucleoside Reverse Transcriptase Inhibitors (NNRTIs)

Nevirapine (Viramune®)

Delavirdine (Rescriptor®)

Efavirenz (Sustiva®)

Fusion Inhibitors

Enfuvirtide (Fuzeon®)

Antibiotics

Penicillin (Pfizerpen®)

Metronidazole (Flagyl®)

Fluoroquinolone Anti-Infectives

Levofloxacin (Levaquin®)

Ofloxacin (Floxin®)

Ciprofloxacin (Cipro®)

Cephalosporin Antibiotics

Ceftriaxone (Rocephin®)

Cefotaxime (Claforan®)

Cefoxitin (Mefoxin®)

Ceftizoxime (Cefizox®)

Cefotetan (Cefotan®)

Macrolide Antibiotics

Clarithromycin (Biaxin)

Azithromycin (Zithromax®)

Erythromycin (E-mycin®)

Tetracyclines

Doxycycline (Vibramycin®)

Tetracycline (Achromycin V®)

Topical Agents

Biological Response Modifiers

Imiquimod (Aldara®)

Antimotitics

Podofilox (Condylox®)

Podophyllin (Podofin®)

Acids

Trichloroacetic acid (TCA®)

Biochlroacetic acid (BCA®)

Scabicides/Pediculocide

Permethrin cream (Elimite®)

Lindane shampoo (Kwell®)

Pyrethrins/piperonyl butoxide (Rid®)

Crotamiton (Eurax®)

GENERAL INFORMATION ABOUT HOW THESE DRUGS WORK

Infections caused by bacteria and parasites are treated, and most can be cured with antibiotics. Infections caused by virus have no known cure. The goal of medication is to keep the symptoms under control. Because there is often a lag time between becoming infected and the appearance of symptoms in some STDs, treatment can be delayed. Regular screenings are very important in order to make sure treatment is begun in a timely manner.

Antiviral drugs are prescribed for different STDs because they work in different ways to prevent the reproduction of particular viruses.

Foscarnet and ganciclovir are prescribed for infections related to the AIDS virus. They interfere with the activity of the enzymes that are necessary for those viruses to reproduce.

Acyclovir, Famciclovir, and Valacyclovir are prescribed for genital herpes. They also interfere with the activity of the enzymes that are necessary for those viruses to reproduce. They do not cure the virus, but they can relieve the pain and inflammation and help the sores heal faster.

Lamivudine and Adefovir are prescribed for hepatitis B. They interfere with the activity of the enzymes that are necessary for those viruses to reproduce. Lamivudine is also prescribed for the HIV virus in high doses and in combination with other medications.

Interferon is used for different types of hepatitis. It acts like the natural interferon that your immune system produces and fights these viruses by slowing, blocking, or changing their function. It might also be prescribed for genital warts.

NRTIs were the first antiretroviral drugs (a type of drug used to treat infections with retroviruses, of which HIV is one) to be developed to treat HIV infection. They interfere with the replication of an HIV enzyme called reverse transcriptase. These medications that work at an early stage of the virus are always used in combination with other drugs.

How HIV Fuses to a Cell
From Project Inform. For more information, contact the National HIV/AIDS Treatment Hotline, 800-822-7422, or visit the website, www.projectinform.org.

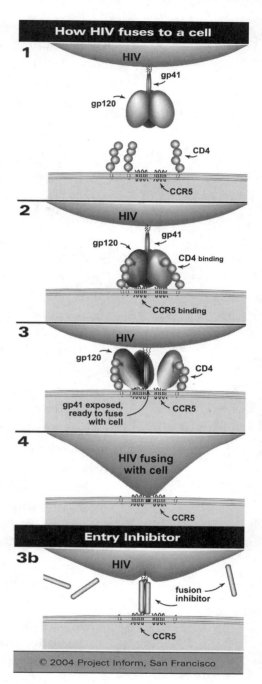

How HIV fuses to a cell

1 · HIV · gp41 · gp120 · CD4 · CCR5

2 · HIV · gp120 · gp41 · CD4 binding · CCR5 binding

3 · HIV · gp120 · CD4 · gp41 exposed, ready to fuse with cell · CCR5

4 · HIV fusing with cell · CCR5

Entry Inhibitor

3b · HIV · fusion inhibitor · CCR5

© 2004 Project Inform, San Francisco

PIs interfere with the replication of the HIV enzyme protease, and they do so at a later stage in the HIV cycle than the NRTIs. Their action on the enzyme protease causes the HIV to become disorganized and noninfectious. These medications are usually included in a combination approach to the disease.

NNRTIs bind to the reverse transcriptase enzyme and prevent it from reproducing. These medications are also usually included in a combination approach to the disease because the HIV virus can become resistant to any of these drugs.

Fusion inhibitors stop the HIV virus from reproducing by preventing it from fusing with healthy cells. This is a newly approved class of drugs that work at the beginning of the HIV cycle. They seem to work on even the most resistant strains of the virus. It keeps the HIV virus from infecting the healthy cell.

Penicillin is given by injection for syphilis. It kills the bacteria by interfering with its cell growth and keeps it from multiplying and spreading.

Metronidazole is thought to destroy bacteria and certain parasites by blocking some of their cell functions, which interferes with their growth and causes them to die. It is prescribed for trichomoniasis.

Fluoroquinolone anti-infectives fight bacteria growth by interfering with an enzyme that is necessary for the bacteria to reproduce. It is prescribed for bacterial infections such as syphilis and gonorrhea.

Cephalosporin antibiotics prevent bacteria from putting up a protective wall to ensure their survival. They are prescribed for bacterial infection such as syphilis, chlamydia, and gonorrhea. They are given by injection.

Microlide antibiotics interfere with the bacteria's ability to make proteins that are necessary for their survival. They are prescribed for bacterial infections such as chancroid and chlamydia and also for some complications of AIDS.

Tetracycline antibiotics interfere with the bacteria's ability to make proteins that are necessary for their survival. They are

> Penicillin was originally discovered by the British bacteriologist Alexander Fleming in September 1928. A culture of staphylococci bacteria growing on an agar medium in a laboratory became contaminated by a mold from the air. The bacteria growing near the mold disappeared. Fleming identified the mold as *Penicillium notatum.* He realized it must have produced an antibiotic substance and he named that substance penicillin. It did not occur to Fleming, at that time, to explore any uses or action of penicillin.
>
> Eleven years later, during World War II, a young University of Virginia student enlisted in the RAF and went to England. He was assigned to work in Fleming's laboratory and started by cleaning it up because there were stacks of dirty dishes and apparatus that appeared to have been there for a long period of time. After the war, when he told of his experiences, the student said he felt the mold would never have grown in the laboratory and spread to the bacteria if the laboratory dishes and apparatus had been cleaned regularly. It was his opinion that penicillin might never have been discovered. Adapted from Alfred Burger, *Drugs and People, Medications, Their History and Origins, and the Way They Act* (Charlottesville: University Press of Virginia, 1986).

prescribed for bacterial infections such as chlamydia and gonorrhea.

Imiquimod, podofilox, podophyllin, biochlroacetic acid, and trichloroacetic acid are prescribed topically for genital warts. They are different types of medications and it is not fully known how they work. It is thought that imiquimod stimulates the skin to produce chemicals to fight genital warts and boost the immune system locally and that podofilox destroys the skin of the wart by inhibiting or preventing cell division. Imiquimod and podofilox can be applied at home. Tricholroacetic acid, biochlroacetic acid, and podophyllin must be applied by a clinician. They burn away the wart from the surface of the skin either with acid or poison.

Scabicides and pediculocides are absorbed into the bodies of the parasites and block their nervous system. This causes paralysis and death. They are prescribed for scabies or crabs.

THE MOST COMMON POSSIBLE SIDE EFFECTS

Antiviral Drugs

- Nausea
- Vomiting
- Irritation at site of ointment application
- Blood in your urine
- Headache
- Abdominal pain
- Lack or loss of strength
- Loss of appetite
- Anxiety
- Confusion
- Fever
- Change in blood count
- Unusual tiredness

BRMs

- Depression
- Muscle ache
- Flu-like symptoms
- Metallic taste in the mouth
- General feeling of discomfort or illness
- Headache
- Loss of appetite
- Nausea
- Vomiting
- Skin rash
- Fatigue

NRTIs

- Nausea
- Vomiting
- Headache

- Loss of appetite
- Diarrhea
- Fever
- Chills
- Rash
- Stomach pain
- Pancreatic inflammation
- Nervous system disturbances
- Sleeplessness
- Weight loss
- Tingling, burning, numbness, or pain in hands, arms, feet, and legs
- Reduced white blood cell counts
- Muscle pain

PIs

- Nausea
- Vomiting
- Diarrhea
- Skin rash
- Dry or itchy skin
- Abdominal pain
- Fatigue
- Headache
- Sleeplessness
- Weakness
- Changes in taste
- Redistribution of body fat
- Elevated cholesterol and triglycerides
- Excess gas
- Tingling feeling

NNRTIs

- Nausea
- Skin rash

- Aches and pains including headache or abdominal pain
- Diarrhea
- Dizziness
- Sleeplessness
- Depression
- Fatigue
- Vomiting
- Poor concentration
- Fever

Fusion Inhibitor

- Local skin reactions and infections at site of injection
- Allergic reaction
- Bacterial pneumonia
- Pain and numbness in feet or legs
- Sleeplessness

Antibiotics

- Nausea
- Vomiting
- Stomach upset or cramps
- Dizziness
- Diarrhea
- Headache
- White patches or sores in the mouth or on the tongue
- Vaginal discharge and itching

Fluoroquinolone Anti-Infectives

- Photosensivity
- Drowsiness
- Nausea
- Abdominal pain

- Diarrhea
- Nervousness
- Constipation

Cephalosporin Antibiotics

- Dizziness
- Headache
- Abdominal pain

Macrolide Antibiotics

- Nausea
- Vomiting
- Abdominal pain
- Diarrhea

Tetracyclines

- Upset stomach
- Nausea
- Vomiting
- Diarrhea
- Skin sensitivity to sun

Topical Biological Response Modifiers

- Irritation at the treated area such as redness, flaking, swelling, or itching

Antimotitics

- Burning, pain, inflammation, or itching of surrounding area

Acids

- Burning of surrounding skin

Scabicides/Pediculocide

◎ Burning or stinging of surrounding skin

OTHER PRECAUTIONS

Antiviral Drugs

◎ These medications have been known to affect pregnancies and can pass into breast milk. Check with your doctor if you are pregnant or nursing.

◎ These medications can cause infertility in men.

BRMs

◎ These medications can add to the effects of alcohol and other central nervous system depressants.

◎ BRMs can increase your chances of getting a different type of infection.

◎ Do not change brands of interferon without checking with your doctor as the dosages and interactions may be different.

NRTIs

◎ These medications have been known to affect pregnancies and can pass into breast milk. Check with your doctor if you are pregnant or nursing.

◎ NRTIs can cause gum infections. See your dentist regularly if you take this type of medication.

◎ Monitor your blood pressure carefully to insure against severe low blood pressure problems.

PIs

◎ This type of medication works best when there is a constant amount in your system. Be sure to follow the directions for dosages very carefully and do not miss any doses.

◎ This medication should be taken with 48oz of water a day and taken on an empty stomach.

- They may decrease the effectiveness of oral contraceptives.
- St. John's Wort has been known to decrease the effectiveness of this type of medication.

NNRTIs

- These medications can add to the effects of alcohol and other central nervous system depressants.
- This type of medication works best when there is a constant amount in your system. Be sure to follow the directions for dosages very carefully and do not miss any doses.
- They may decrease the effectiveness of oral contraceptives.
- Antacid medication can affect the absorption of this type of medication.

Fusion Inhibitor

- This type of medication is too new to know about any long-term precautions.

Antibiotics

- Penicillin is the first line of treatment for syphilis. Make sure you are not allergic to penicillin. If so, your doctor can work with you to find another effective treatment.
- Penicillin can interfere with the action of oral contraceptives.
- Penicillin can be destroyed by fruit juices and carbonated drinks. Take pills with still water.
- You may develop an itchy rash with penicillin that is not a true allergic reaction. Check all rashes with your doctor.

Fluoroquinolone Anti-Infectives

- These medications can make you drowsy or dizzy. Make sure you know how they affect you before you do anything that requires your full alertness.
- Some strains of gonorrhea are resistant to this type of antibiotic.

Cephalosporin Antibiotics

◎ Cephalosporin antibiotics are chemically related to penicillin. If you are allergic to penicillin, you may not be able to take cephalosporin antibiotics.

◎ These medications can add to the effects of alcohol and other central nervous system depressants.

Macrolide Antibiotics

◎ These medications may pass into breast milk. You may want to consider bottle-feeding if you are taking this type of medication.

Tetracyclines

◎ Some prescription oral antibiotics may reduce the effectiveness of oral contraceptives. You will need to use an additional form of birth control if you are taking these medications.

◎ Antibiotics can also increase the effects of caffeine.

◎ Antacids can reduce the effectiveness of these oral antibiotics since they bind the oral antibiotics in the intestines.

◎ These medications have been known to affect pregnancies and can pass into breast milk. Check with your doctor if you are pregnant or nursing.

Topical Biological Response Modifiers

◎ Imiquimod can weaken external birth control methods such as condoms and diaphragms.

Antimotitics

◎ Podophyllum is a poison and must be kept away from your eyes and mouth.

◎ Large amounts of podophyllum can cause nerve damage.

Acids

◎ These are for external warts only.

Scabicides/Pediculocide

◎ **Lindane treatments should be limited to the prescribed four-minute period to ensure against potentially harmful central nervous system complications.**

◎ **Lindane is a poison and must be kept away from your eyes and mouth.**

◎ **These medications have been known to affect pregnancies and can pass into breast milk. Check with your doctor if you are pregnant or nursing.**

THE BOTTOM LINE

The only way to prevent getting STDs is to abstain from sex. Other alternatives are to limit your number of sex partners, ask your partner if he or she has been tested for STDs, and always make sure you use a condom when you engage in any type of sexual activity. (Be aware that condoms are not 100 percent safe against contracting STDs.)

If you are sexually active, you should have frequent medical checkups to make sure you are not infected and in need of medication.

It was once thought that spermicides would help prevent STDs. Research now shows that that frequent use of N-9, a spermicide contraceptive, can actually make you more susceptible to STDs because it can cause lesions in the vagina and the rectum that provide an entry point for infections.

Some types of STDs can become resistant to the drugs used to treat them. Work closely with your doctor to make sure the medication you are using is the right one.

Antiviral drugs and antibiotics can cause pregnancy and nursing problems. They can also cause infertility. STDs have similar side effects. You should talk with your doctor to weigh the risks of the medications versus the disease.

This may be an embarrassing condition, but the health risks are great. Make sure you have a good relationship with your doctor or other medical professional so you can talk with her or him about everything.

If topical treatments do not work for genital warts, surgery is a possibility. Surgery might include:

- Freezing the area with liquid nitrogen (cryosurgery)
- Burning the area with electricity (electrocautery)
- Receiving laser treatments

18 Tourette Syndrome (TS)

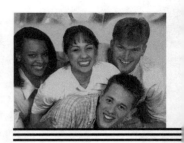

Tourette Syndrome (TS) is a neurological condition that is characterized by uncontrollable movements and noises, called tics, which can come and go over time. You also may exhibit obsessive-compulsive behaviors, an intense uncontrollable need to do something repeatedly.

THE MOST COMMON PRESCRIPTION MEDICATIONS

Antipsychotic Drugs (Neuroleptics)

Haloperidol (Haldol®)

Pimozide (Orap®)

Fluphenazine (Prolixin®)

Risperidone (Risperdal®)

Antihypertensive Drugs

Clonidine (Catapres®)

Guanfacine (Tenex®)

Antianxiety Medications

Clonazepam (Klonopin®)

Neurotoxin

Botulinum Toxin (Botox)

GENERAL INFORMATION ABOUT HOW THESE DRUGS WORK

The specific cause of TS is not fully known. The research indicates that there is an imbalance of the neurotransmitters dopamine, serotonin, and norepinephrine. The medications do not cure the disorder. They only help specific symptoms. Determining which medication to use is based on which symptoms are being targeted and what the side effects are.

Antipsychotic drugs (neuroleptics) appear to act on the neurotransmitters in your brain, but research to date has not been able to determine exactly how this happens. They are thought to work on different combinations of neurotransmitters and affect the amount of these chemicals available to the cells in your brain and how the nerves communicate with each other. They appear to block certain receptors on the nerves so that they are not activated. This does not cure the tics, but it can affect the number and severity of them.

Antihypertensives stimulate nerve endings in the brain by affecting the neurotransmitter norepinephrine. Doing this relaxes the blood vessels so blood can flow through more easily.

Antianxiety medications are central nervous system depressants. They slow down your nervous system by helping gamma-aminobutyric acid (GABA) inhibit activity in some of the nerves in the brain.

Botox, injected in the muscle involved in the tics, may decrease the involuntary movement and the urge to move.

THE MOST COMMON POSSIBLE SIDE EFFECTS

Antipsychotic Drugs (Neuroleptics)

- Drowsiness
- Blurred vision
- Faintness or dizziness
- Restlessness
- Unusual posture or walk
- Mild stiffness or rigidity
- Shaking or sudden jerky movements

- Constipation
- Decreased sweating
- Nausea
- Headache
- Drowsiness
- Behavior or mood changes
- Sleeplessness
- Dry mouth
- Sexual changes
- Sore breasts
- Agitation or anxiety

Antihypertensive Drugs

- Dry mouth
- Drowsiness
- Dizziness
- Constipation
- Tiredness

Antianxiety Medications

- Drowsiness
- Unsteadiness
- Dizziness
- Lightheadedness
- Slurred speech

Neurotoxin

- Weakness in the muscle where it was injected
- Injection site reactions such as pain and bleeding

OTHER PRECAUTIONS

Antipsychotic Drugs (Neuroleptics)

- These medications have been known to affect pregnancies and can pass into breast milk. Check with your doctor if you are pregnant or nursing.

◎ These medications can make you drowsy. Make sure you know how they affect you before you do anything that requires your full alertness.

◎ If a dry mouth is one of the side effects you experience, be alert to the possibility of dental problems.

◎ These medications can make your skin more sensitive to the sun and changes in body temperature. Make sure you take proper precautions when in the sun and avoid tanning booths and sun lamps as well as saunas and hot tubs.

Antihypertensive Drugs

◎ There have been incidences of impaired sexual function in some people taking clonidine.

◎ Clonidine and guanfacine are used for high blood pressure and they reduce heart rate. Do not take other medications that are designed to reduce heart rate without discussing this with your doctor.

Antianxiety Medications

◎ These medications are generally prescribed for short periods of time because you can develop a tolerance to them. That means that you will have to stop taking the medication or the dosage will have to be increased.

◎ They also can become habit forming if taken for a long period of time. Be alert to signs that this happening.

◎ These medications have been known to affect pregnancies and can pass into breast milk. Check with your doctor if you are pregnant or nursing.

◎ These medications can add to the effects of alcohol and other central nervous system depressants.

Neurotoxin

◎ Long-term effects of this treatment are unknown.

THE BOTTOM LINE

Many people with TS do not use medications. You and your doctor need to work closely together to determine if your symptoms are so disruptive to your life that medications might be worth a try.

You need to weigh the side effects of the medications with how severe your symptoms are when you are not on medications. You also need to think about your lifestyle and how the symptoms and the side effects will change what you do. Driving a car, drinking with your friends, and planning a family are serious issues that must be considered in any course of treatment.

You might have some other problem, such as ADHD, as well as TS. Make sure your doctors know about all difficulties you are having and all medications you are taking. There are some ADHD medications that should not be taken if you have tics. Some medications can be used to treat more than one problem. You need to make sure you are taking the right medications for all of your symptoms.

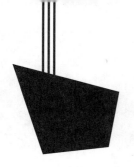

Glossary:
Terms Related to
Medications and
Conditions Included
in This Book

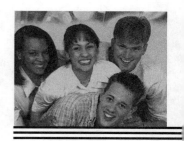

504 plan: an accommodation plan that will provide you with any necessary changes in your school day due to illness or disability

absence seizure: a type of seizure that is a momentary break in consciousness and may be characterized by eye-blinking or twitching, also known as a petit mal seizure

adolescent medicine: doctors who specialize in treating teenagers

AIDS: *See* human immunodeficiency virus/acquired immune deficiency syndrome (HIV/AIDS)

allergen: a foreign body that produces an allergic reaction

alpha-glucosidase inhibitors: medications used to treat type 2 diabetes by slowing the breakdown of the complex sugars into glucose

aminosalicylates: medications to treat the inflammation associated with Crohn's disease

amygdala: a small structure deep inside the brain that coordinates your body's fear response

analgesics: medications that control pain

anaphylactic shock: a severe and sometimes life-threatening reaction to a foreign body such as an allergen, food, or drug that results in respiratory problems, fainting, or cardiac arrest

androgen: a male sex hormone

anemia: a condition where your blood does not have enough red blood cells

anorexia nervosa: an intense fear of being fat so that you hardly eat at all

antibacterials: medications that fight bacteria

antibiotic: a medication that can kill or inhibit the growth of bacteria

antibody: a protein that is produced by your immune system in response to a toxic substance and that acts against that toxin

anticholinergics: a type of drug that blocks the effects of the naturally occurring body chemical acetylcholine and prevents your nasal membranes from producing too much mucus as one of its functions

anticonvulsant: a medication used to treat, stop, or prevent seizures

antidepressant: a prescription drug designed to minimize the symptoms of depression

antihistamine: medication that can reduce swelling, inflammation, and other effects of an allergic reaction

antihypertensives: medications that are used in treating high blood pressure

antimalarials: medications traditionally used to fight malaria, but that have been found to have an anti-inflammatory effect in fighting the symptoms of lupus and a variety of other diseases

antimitotic: inhibits or prevents cell division

antinausea medications: medications used to treat nausea and vomiting

antiretroviral: a type of drug used to treat infections with retroviruses like HIV

antiviral drugs: medications used to treat virus-related sexually transmitted diseases, including HIV, because they keep the viruses from reproducing

ataxia: a disorder where you are unable to coordinate voluntary muscle movements

atypical antidepressants: medications for depression and anxiety that do not fit well into any other major medication category

azaspirones: medication used to treat anxiety with less potential for addiction than other medications for anxiety

BED: *See* binge eating disorder (BED)

benzodiazepines: a medication that has a tranquilizing or sedative effect

beta-blockers: drugs that block the activity of a beta-receptor and decrease heart rate, lower blood pressure, and prevent migraine headaches

biguanides: medications used to treat diabetes that lower the amount of glucose made by your liver

binge eating disorder (BED): repeated episodes of compulsive overeating without purging

biologic response modifiers (BRMs): medications given by injection to block the body's biological response

bipolar disorder: a brain disorder that causes unusual, severe shifts in mood, energy, and ability to function. This is also known as manic depression.

blackhead: a comedo, or plugged hair follicle, that is open on the skin and the top appears to be black

BRMs: *See* biologic response modifiers (BRMs)

bronchial tubes: airways to the lungs

bronchodilators: a drug that relaxes the bronchial muscles and expands the air passages

bulimia nervosa: an intense fear of being fat where you eat large amounts of food, so you get rid of it by vomiting (purging) or taking laxatives

calcium channel blockers: blood pressure lowering medication that is used to treat migraines because it helps blood vessels relax

cataracts: a clouding of the lens of the eye that blocks the passage of light into the area for sight

central nervous system depressants: substances, including medications, that act on your brain and spinal column that may cause drowsiness

chlamydia: a sexually transmitted disease caused by bacteria

comedo: a hair follicle that is plugged with sebum, hair cells, and often bacteria

complimentary treatments: herbal treatments that appear to help a particular condition, but that have not been tested by the FDA for that application

corticosteroids: prescription drugs that are used to reduce inflammation

COX-2 inhibitors: drugs for pain and inflammation that have fewer gastrointestinal side effects than traditional nonsteroidal anti-inflammatory drugs because they do not block the hormone that helps maintain the protective lining in your stomach

crabs (pubic lice): a sexually transmitted infestation of crab lice

Crohn's disease: an inflammation in the small intestine that can cause chronic pain and diarrhea

cryosurgery: freezing the area with liquid nitrogen

decongestant: a drug that relieves congestion of the mucus membranes

dialysis: an artificial filtering system that does the filtering job that the kidneys can no longer do

dilate: expand

disease-modifying antirheumatic drugs (DMARDs): drugs that suppress the immune cells that are responsible for inflammation

diuretics: a drug that increases the output of urine

DMARDs: *See* disease-modifying antirheumatic drugs (DMARDs)

dopamine: a neurotransmitter in the brain that regulates nerve activity

drug interactions: increased side effects that occur when two drugs interact, causing some type of change in the action of either drug

dysthymic depression: mild depression that appears to continue for a long period of time

electrocautery: Burning an area with electricity for medical purposes

electrolytes: substances in the body, such as sodium, potassium, calcium, or bicarbonate, that are vital for the metabolic processes of your body

epilepsy: an underlying disease of the brain that is manifest by recurring seizures

ergot alkaloids: medications used to treat migraines that narrow the dilated blood vessels and reduce the inflammation associated with the dilation

erythropoietin: a hormonal substance that stimulates the formation of red blood cells

fusion inhibitor: a new class of drug that stops the HIV virus from reproducing by preventing it from fusing with healthy cells

GABA: *See* gamma-aminobutyric acid (GABA)

gamma-aminobutyric acid (GABA): a neurotransmitter in the brain that regulates nerve activity in the brain

generalized tonic-clonic (grand mal) seizures: seizures that involve the entire body and are usually characterized by muscle rigidity, violent muscle contractions, and loss of consciousness

generic: relating to the characteristics of a whole group

genital warts: a viral sexually transmitted disease that is characterized by growths or bumps in and around the genital area

GI problems: problems with your gastrointestinal system

glucose: the main fuel for your body

gonorrhea: a bacterial sexually transmitted disease that can grow and multiply in warm mucus areas of the body and can lead to serious, permanent problems if not treated

hair follicle: the tiny shaft in the skin through which a hair grows and where sebum is excreted from glands to the surface of the skin

hepatitis B: a viral sexually transmitted disease that can cause severe liver problems and death

histamines: a compound that is released during an allergic reaction and that causes symptoms such as watery eyes, itching, and runny nose

HIV: *See* human immunodeficiency virus/acquired immune deficiency syndrome (HIV/AIDS)

human immunodeficiency virus/acquired immune deficiency syndrome (HIV/AIDS): a sexually transmitted disease caused by a retrovirus that destroys your body's ability to fight infection

hormonal therapies: medications to treat acne that contain a female hormone to block the affects of male hormones

hormone: the product of a cell that affects how the cell functions

hirsutism: excessive growth and distribution of hair in a male pattern, especially in women

immunomodulators: a chemical agent that modifies how your immune system functions

immunotherapy: a treatment against a disease by inducing immunity to the disease

insulin: a protein hormone, which is synthesized in your pancreas, that promotes utilization of glucose by the cells

lesions: physical changes in body tissue; in acne, it is a physical change in the skin caused by the disease in the hair follicle

leukotriene: a chemical that occurs naturally in the body and can bind to other cells causing inflammation

lubricants: creams, lotions, and ointments that you apply to your skin to decrease moisture loss and dryness

mast cells: tissue cells that make and release histamines and other causes of inflammation

metabolized: processed by your body and made available for its use

monoamine oxidase: an enzyme in your body that breaks down certain neurotransmitters

monoclonal antibody: a protein that is developed to mimic the body's own antibodies in order to suppress abnormal cell changes that would result in disease

mood stabilizers: medications that increase the amount of neurotransmitter available to your cells and that have a stabilizing effect on your mood

myoclonic seizures: a brief, single or multiple, irregular muscle contraction that may or may not include a loss of consciousness.

narcolepsy: brief uncontrollable episodes of deep sleep

narcotic: a drug that dulls the senses, relieves pain, and induces drowsiness

nebulizer: a way to deliver medication in a mist

nephritis: an inflammation of the filtering units of your kidneys

nephrosis: damage to the filtering units of your kidneys

neuroleptic (antipsychotic): a powerful tranquilizer used to treat psychoses

neurons: cells in your nervous system that send and receive impulses

neurotoxin: a potentially poisonous substance that inhibits, damages, or destroys tissues and cells of the nervous system

neurotransmitter: a chemical that carries the nerve impulse from one nerve cell to another

noncomedogenic: cosmetics that do not clog pores

nonsteroidal anti-inflammatory drugs (NSAIDs): drugs that work by blocking your body's production of specific hormones and chemicals that contribute to inflammation and pain

nonstimulant: a medication to treat ADHD that reduces the reabsorption of norepinephrine by the nerves and leaves more of it available to communicate with other nerves

norepinephrine: a neurotransmitter linked to mood, emotion, and mental state

NRTIs: *See* nucleoside analogue reverse transcriptase inhibitors (NRTIs)

NSAIDs: *See* nonsteroidal anti-inflammatory drugs (NSAIDs)

nucleoside analogue reverse transcriptase inhibitors (NRTIs): the first antiretroviral drugs to be developed to treat HIV infection, interfering with the replication of an HIV enzyme called reverse transcriptase

nystagmus: a rapid, involuntary shaking of the eyeballs

obsessive-compulsive behaviors: recurrent and persistent ideas and thoughts that get in the way of everyday activities and/or rituals and repetitive activities that also get in the way of normal activities

partial seizures: seizures that start in one part of the brain and may include weakness, numbness, unusual smells and tastes, and muscle twitching without loss of consciousness, or may be complex with some of the same symptoms as above but with changes in consciousness and the ability to interact appropriately with the environment

pelvic inflammatory disease (PID): an infection in the female reproductive tract that can lead to infertility

PID: *See* pelvic inflammatory disease (PID)

PIs: *See* protease inhibitors (PIs)

prophylactic: something used to prevent disease

prostaglandins: hormone-like substances that are found in many parts of the body and that stimulate cells to act

protease inhibitors (PIs): medications for AIDS/HIV that interfere with the replication of the HIV enzyme protease

psychotherapy: treatment of mental or emotional disorders by communication with a qualified therapist

psychotropic drugs: drugs that affect the mind through action on the nervous system

purging: inducing evacuation of your bowels as with laxatives

retinoids: a form of vitamin A

retroviral infections: the presence of viruses that grow by inserting their genetic material in the chromosome of a host's cells and are spread by that host's cells

reverse transcriptase: an enzyme that copies the genetic material of the HIV virus and instructs infected cells to make additional copies of the virus

St. John's Wort: an herbal product sold as a treatment for depression

scabicides: a drug that destroys the mites that cause scabies

scabies: a disease caused by parasitic mites that is transmitted through contact

sebaceous glands: the glands in the skin that produce sebum

sebum: the oily substance that is produced by sebaceous glands and is excreted to the surface of your skin

selective serotonin reuptake inhibitors (SSRIs): substance that keeps the neurotransmitter serotonin from being absorbed by your cells and keeps it in the spaces surrounding the nerve endings of the cells in your brain

serotonin: a neurotransmitter in the brain that regulates nerve activity in the brain

side effect: the unwanted result of a medication that you are taking for a particular condition

spermicides: a substance used as a birth control device designed to kill sperm

SSRIs: *See* selective serotonin reuptake inhibitors (SSRIs)

steroids: a large family of substances including sex hormones and other elements essential for normal body function and maintenance

stimulants: a group of medications that increase alertness and physical activity

substance P: a neurotransmitter that is associated with the transmission of pain and may be present at an increased level in those with depression and anxiety disorders

sulfa: *See* sulfonamide (sulfa)

sulfonamide (sulfa): a medication that fights the growth of bacteria

sympathomimetic agents: medications that mimic your body's automatic response to fight stress or an emergency situation. They affect a variety of body functions

syphilis: a sexually transmitted disease caused by the bacterium Treponema pallidum that shows up first as single or multiple sores and may proceed to more serious symptoms and possibly death if not treated

thiazide: medication that is used to remove water from your body but that also removes potassium and magnesium along with the water

thiazolidinediones (glitazones): medications for diabetes that make your body more sensitive to insulin and make the insulin work better

tics: uncontrollable movements and noises

topical medication: medication that is applied to your skin

trichomoniasis: a sexually transmitted disease caused by the parasite Trichomonas vaginalis

triptans: medications developed specifically for migraines that narrow the blood vessels that become wider during an attack

tyramine: a substance that is found in some foods such as aged cheese and wine that can interact with MAOIs, causing dangerous side effects

ulcerative colitis: a disease that causes inflammation and sores in the lining of the large intestine

vasoconstrictors: medications for migraines that help counteract the painful dilation stage of the headache by constricting the dilated blood vessels

whitehead: a comedo, or plugged, hair follicle that is under the skin and appears as a skin-colored bump

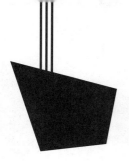

List of Medications
by Generic Name

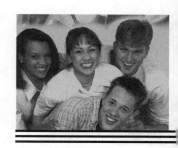

too much? Do you feel guilty things that aren't your fault? I

Generic Name	One Brand Name	Type	Used for
Abacavir	Ziagen®	NRTI	STD
Acarbose	Precose®	Alpha-glucosidase inhibitor	Diabetes
Acetaminophen	Tylenol®	Analgesic	JRA; Migraine
Acetaminophen/Butalbital	Phrenilin®	Analgesic/Sedative	Migraine
Acetaminophen/Butalbital/ Caffeine	Esgic®	Analgesic/Sedative	Migraine
Acetaminophen/Codeine	Tylenol with Codeine®	Analgesic/Narcotic	JRA; Migraine
Acyclovir	Zovirax®	Antiviral	STD
Adalimumab	Humira®	BRM	JRA
Adapalene	Differin®	Topical Retinoid	Acne
Adefovir	Hepsera®	Antiviral	STD
Albuterol	Proventil®	Inhaled Bronchodilator	Asthma
Albuterol Sulfate and Ipratroprium Bromide	Combivent®	Inhaled Bronchodilators	Asthma
Almotriptan	Axert®	Triptan	Migraine
Alprazolam	Xanax®	Benzodiazepine	Anxiety
Amiloride	Midamor®	Diuretic	Kidney Disease
Amitriptyline	Elavil®	Tricyclic Antidepressant	Anxiety; Depression; Migraine

Amprenavir	Agenerase®	Protease Inhibitor	STD
Aspart	NovoLog®	Quick-acting Insulin	Diabetes
Aspirin	Arthritis Pain Formula®	Salicylate/NSAID	JRA; Migraine
Aspirin/Acetaminophen/Caffeine	Excedrin Migraine®	Analgesic	Migraine
Aspirin/Butalbital/Caffeine	Fiorinal®	Analgesic/Sedative	Migraine
Aspirin/Codeine	Empirin with Codeine®	Analgesic/Narcotic	Migraine
Atenolol	Tenormin®	Beta-Blocker	Migraine
Atomoxetine	Strattera®	Nonstimulant	ADHD
Azathioprine	Imuran®	Immunosuppressant	JRA; IBD; Lupus
Azelaic Acid Lotion	Azelex®	Topical Antibacterial	Acne
Azelastine	Astelin®	Antihistamine	Allergies
Azelastine	Optivar®	Antihistamine Eye Drops	Allergies
Azithromycin	Zithromax®	Antibiotic	STD
Balsalazide Disodium	Colazal®	Aminosalicylate	IBD
Beclomethasone	Beconase AQ®	Corticosteroid—Nasal Spray	Allergies

Beclomethasone	Vanceril®	Corticosteroid—Inhaled	Asthma
Bendroflumethiazide	Naturetin®	Diuretic	Kidney Disease
Benzoyl Peroxide	Clearasil®	OTC Acne Medication	Acne
Benzoyl Peroxide	Clearasil Maximum Strength®	Topical Antibacterial	Acne
Betamethasone Dipropionate	Diprolene®	Topical Corticosteroid	Eczema; Lupus
Biochlroacetic acid	BCA®	Topical Acid	STD
Botulinum Toxin	Botox®	Neuromuscular Blocker	Migraine; Tourette
Budesonide	Pulmicort®	Corticosteroid—Inhaled	Asthma
Budesonide	Rhinocort®	Corticosteroid—Nasal Spray	Allergies
Bumetanide	Bumex®	Diuretic	Kidney Disease
Bupropion	Wellbutrin®	Atypical Antidepressant	Depression
Buspirone	BuSpar®	Azaspirone	Anxiety
Capsaicin	Zostrix®	Analgesic/Topical	JRA
Carbamazepine	Tegretol®	Mood Stabilizer/Anticonvulsant	Depression; Seizures
Cefotaxime	Claforan®	Antibiotic	STD
Cefotetan	Cefotan®	Antibiotic	STD
Cefoxitin	Mefoxin®	Antibiotic	STD

Ceftizoxime	Antibiotic	STD
Ceftriaxone	Antibiotic	STD
Celecoxib	COX-2 Inhibitor/NSAID	JRA; Lupus
Cetirizine	Antihistamine	Allergies
Chloroquine	Antimalarial	Lupus
Chlorothiazide	Diuretic	Kidney Disease
Chlorpheniramine	Antihistamine OTC	Allergies
Choline and Magnesium Salicylate	Salicylate/NSAID	JRA
Choline Salicylate	Salicylate/NSAID	JRA
Ciprofloxacin	Antibiotic	IBD; STD
Citalopram	SSRI	Anxiety; Depression; Eating Disorders
Clarithromycin	Antibiotic	STD
Clemastine	Antihistamine OTC	Allergies
Clindamycin	Topical Antibiotic	Acne
Clobetasol Propionate	Topical Corticosteroid	Eczema; Lupus
Clomipramine	Tricyclic Antidepressant	Anxiety
Clonazepam	Benzodiazepine	Anxiety; Seizures; Tourette
Clonidine	Antihypertensive	Tourette

Cefizox®		
Rocephin®		
Celebrex®		
Zyrtec®		
Aralen®		
Diuril®		
Chlor-Trimeton®		
Tricosal®		
Arthropan®		
Cipro®		
Celexa®		
Biaxin®		
Tavist®		
Cleocin T-ge®		
Cormax®		
Anafranil®		
Klonopin®		
Catapres®		

Cromolyn Sodium	NasalCrom®	Mast Cell Stabilizer—Inhalant	Allergies; Asthma
Crotamiton	Eurax®	Scabicide	STD
Cyclophosphamide	Cytoxan®	Immunosuppressant	Lupus
Cyclosporine	Sandimmune®	Immunosuppressant	JRA; Eczema; IBD; Lupus
Cyproheptadine	Periactin®	Antihistamine	Migraine
d-Penicillamine	Cuprimine®	Immunosuppressant	JRA
Delavirdine	Rescriptor®	NNRTI	STD
Desipramine	Norpramin®	Tricyclic Antidepressant	ADHD; Depression
Desloratadine	Clarinex®	Antihistamine	Allergies
Desonide	DesOwen®	Topical Corticosteroid	Eczema
Dexamethasone	Decadron®	Corticosteroid	JRA; Asthma; Lupus
Dexmethylphenidate	Focalin®	Stimulant	ADHD
Dextro-Amphetamine	Dexedrine®	Stimulant	ADHD
Dextro-Amphetamine and Amphetamine	Adderall®	Stimulant	ADHD
Diazepam	Valium®	Benzodiazepine	Anxiety; Seizures
Diclofenac	Voltaren®	NSAID	JRA; Lupus
Didanosine	Videx®	NRTI	STD
Diflunisal	Dolobid®	NSAID	Lupus

Dihydroergotamine	DHE-45®	Injectable Ergot Alkaloid	Migraine
Dihydroergotamine	Migranal®	Ergot Alkaloid—Nasal	Migraine
Diltiazem	Cardizem®	Calcium Channel Blocker	Migraine
Diphenhydramine	Benadryl®	Antihistamine OTC	Allergies
Divalproex	Depakote®	Anticonvulsant	Migraine
Doxepin	Sinequan®	Tricyclic Antidepressant	Migraine
Doxycycline	Vibramycin®	Antibiotic	Acne; STD
Efavirenz	Sustiva®	NNRTI	STD
Emedastine	Emadine®	Antihistamine Eye Drops	Allergies
Enfuvirtide	Fuzeon®	Fusion Inhibitor	STD
Epinephrine	Epipen®	Sympathomimetic Agent	Allergies
Ergotamine	Ergostat®	Ergot Alkaloid	Migraine
Ergotamine/Caffeine	Wigraine®	Ergot Alkaloid	Migraine
Erythromycin	E-mycin®	Antibiotic	Acne; STD
Erythromycin	Staticin®	Topical Antibiotic	Acne
Estrogen Contraceptives	Ortho Tri-Cyclen®	Hormonal Therapy	Acne
Etanercept	Enbrel®	BRM	JRA
Ethacrynic Acid	Edecrin®	Diuretic	Kidney Disease
Ethosuximide	Zarontin®	Anticonvulsant	Seizures

Etodolac	NSAID	Lupus
Famciclovir	Antiviral	STDs
Felbamate	Anticonvulsant	Seizure
Fexofenadine	Antihistamine	Allergies
Fexofenadine and Pseudoephedrine	Decongestant/ Antihistamine	Allergies
Flunisolide	Corticosteroid—Inhaled	Asthma
Flunisolide	Corticosteroid—Nasal Spray	Allergies
Fluocinolone	Topical Corticosteroid	Lupus
Fluocinonide	Topical Corticosteroid	Eczema; Lupus
Fluoxetine	SSRI	Anxiety; Depression; Eating Disorders; Migraine
Fluphenazine	Neuroleptic	Tourette
Flurandrenolide	Topical Corticosteroid	Eczema
Fluticasone	Corticosteroid—Nasal Spray	Allergies
Fluticasone	Corticosteroid—Inhaled	Asthma
Fluvoxamine	SSRI	Anxiety; Depression; Eating Disorders

Lodine®		
Famvir®		
Felbatol®		
Allegra®		
Allegra D®		
Aerobid®		
Nasalide®		
Synalar®		
Lidex®		
Prozac®		
Prolixin®		
Cordan®		
Flonase®		
Flovent®		
Luvox®		

Formoterol	Foradil®	Inhaled Bronchodilator	Asthma
Foscarnet	Foscavir®	Antiviral	STDs
Frovatriptan	Frova®	Triptan	Migraine
Furosemide	Lasix®	Diuretic	Kidney Disease
Gabapentin	Neurontin®	Mood Stabilizer/Anticonvulsant	Anxiety; Depression; Migraine; Seizures
Ganciclovir	Cytovene®	Antiviral	STDs
Glargine	Lantus®	Peakless Insulin	Diabetes
Glycolic Acid	Alpha Hydroxy®	OTC Acne Medication	Acne
Gold	Myochrisine®	DMARD	JRA
Guanfacine	Tenex®	Antihypertensive	Tourette
Halobetasol	Ultravate®	Topical Corticosteroid	Lupus
Haloperidol	Haldol®	Neuroleptic	Tourette
Hydrochlorothiazide	Esidrix®	Diuretic	Kidney Disease
Hydrocodone/ Acetaminophen	Vicodin®	Analgesic	JRA
Hydrocortisone	Hydrocortone®	Corticosteroid	Asthma; Eczema
Hydrocortisone	Dermacort®	Topical Corticosteroid	Eczema; Lupus
Hydroxychloroquine	Plaquenil®	Antimalarial DMARD	Lupus; JRA
Ibuprofen	Advil®	NSAID	JRA; Lupus; Migraine

Imipramine	Tofranil®	Tricyclic Antidepressant	ADHD; Depression
Imiquimod	Aldara®	Topical BRM	STD
Indinavir	Crixivan®	Protease Inhibitor	STD
Indomethacin	Indocin®	NSAID	Lupus
Infliximab	Remicade®	BRM	JRA; IBD
Insulin Regular	Humulin R®	Short-acting Insulin	Diabetes
Interferon-alpha	Intron A®	BRM	STD
Ipratropium	Atrovent®	Inhaled Bronchodilator	Asthma
Isometheptene/ Acetaminophen/ Dichloralphenazone	Midrin®	Analgesic/sedative	Migraine
Isotretinoin	Accutane®	Systemic Retinoid	Acne
Ketoprofen	Orudis®	NSAID	Lupus; Migraine
Ketorolac	Acular®	NSAID/Eye Drops	Allergies
Lamivudine	Epivir®	Antiviral	STD
Lamotrigine	Lamictal®	Mood Stabilizer/ Anticonvulsant	Depression Seizures
Leflunomide	Arava®	DMARD	JRA
Lente Insulin	Humulin L®	Intermediate-acting Insulin	Diabetes
Levalbuterol	Xopenex®	Inhaled Bronchodilator	Asthma

Generic Name	Brand Name	Classification	Use
Levetiracetam	Keppra®	Anticonvulsant	Seizures
Levocabastine	Livostin®	Antihistamine Eye Drops	Allergies
Levofloxacin	Levaquin®	Antibiotic	STD
Lindane	Kwell®	Pediculocide Shampoo	STD
Lispro	Humalog®	Quick-acting Insulin	Diabetes
Lithium	Eskalith®	Mood Stabilizer	Depression
Lodoxamide	Alomide®	Mass Cell Stabilizer/Eye Drops	Allergies
Lopinavir/Ritonavir	Kaletra®	Protease Inhibitor	STD
Loratadine	Claritin®	Antihistamine OTC	Allergies
Lorazepam	Ativan®	Benzodiazepine	Anxiety Seizures
Meloxicam	Mobic®	NSAID	Lupus
Menthol	Eucalyptamint®	Analgesic/Topical	JRA
Mercaptopurine (6-MP)	Purinethol®	Immunosuppressant	IBD
Mesalamine	Asacol®	Aminosalicylate	IBD
Metformin	Glucophage®	Biguanide	Diabetes
Methotrexate	Rheumatrex®	DMARD/Immunosuppressant	JRA; IBD; Lupus
Methyclothiazide	Enduron®	Diuretic	Kidney Disease

Generic Name	Brand Name	Type	Use
Methyl Salicylate	BenGay®	Analgesic/Topical	JRA
Methyl Salicylate and Menthol	IcyHot®	Analgesic/Topical	JRA
Methylphenidate	Concerta®	Extended-Release Stimulant	ADHD
Methylphenidate	Ritalin®	Short-acting Stimulant	ADHD
Methylprednisolone	Medrol®	Corticosteroid	Asthma; Eczema; IBS; Lupus
Metoclopramide	Reglan®	Antinausea	Migraine
Metoprolol	Lopressor®	Beta-Blocker	Migraine
Metronidazole	Flagyl®	Antibiotic	IBD; STD
Miglitol	Glyset®	Alpha-glucosidase Inhibitors	Diabetes
Minocycline	Minocin®	Antibiotic	Acne
Mirtazapine	Remeron®	Atypical Antidepressant	Depression
Mometasone	Elocon®	Topical Corticosteroid	Eczema
Mometasone	Nasonex®	Corticosteroid—Nasal Spray	Allergies
Montelukast	Singulair®	Leukotriene Modifier	Allergies; Asthma
Nabumetone	Relafen®	NSAID	Lupus
Nadolol	Corgard®	Beta-Blocker	Migraine
Naphazoline and Pheniramine	Visine-A®	Decongestant/Antihistamine Eye Drops	Allergies

Naproxen	Aleve®	NSAID	JRA; Migraine; Lupus
Naratriptan	Amerge®	Triptan	Migraine
Nedocromil	Alocril®	Mass Cell Stabilizer	Allergies; Asthma
Nefazodone	Serzone®	Atypical Antidepressant	Anxiety; Depression
Nelfinavir	Viracept®	Protease Inhibitor	STD
Nevirapine	Viramune®	NNRTI	STD
Nifedipine	Adalat®	Calcium Channel Blocker	Migraine
Nortriptyline	Pamelor®	Tricyclic Antidepressant	ADHD; Depression; Migraine
NPH Insulin	Humulin N®	Short-acting Insulin	Diabetes
NPH Insulin and Insulin	Humulin 50/50®	Combination Insulin	Diabetes
Ofloxacin	Floxin®	Antibiotic	STD
Olopatadine	Patanol®	Antihistamine Eye Drops	Allergies
Omalizumab	Xolair®	Monoclonal Antibody	Asthma
Oxaprozin	Daypro®	NSAID	Lupus
Oxcarbazepine	Trileptal®	Anticonvulsant	Seizures
Oxycodone/Acetaminophen	Percocet®	Analgesic/Narcotic	JRA; Migraine
Oxycodone/Aspirin	Percodan®	Analgesic/Narcotic	Migraine
Oxymetazoline	Afrin®	Decongestant Nasal Spray	Allergies
		OTC	

Generic	Brand	Class	Use
Paroxetine	Paxil®	SSRI	Anxiety; Depression; Eating Disorders; Migraine
Pemoline	Cylert®	Stimulant	ADHD
Penicillin	Pfizerpen®	Antibiotic	STD
Permethrin Cream	Elimite®	Scabicide	STD
Phenelzine	Nardil®	MAOI	Anxiety
Phenobarbital	Solfoton®	Anticonvulsant	Seizures
Phenylephrine	Neo-Synephrine®	Decongestant Nasal Spray OTC	Allergies
Phenytoin	Dilantin®	Anticonvulsant	Seizures
Pimecrolimus	Elidel Cream®	Topical Immunomodulator	Eczema
Pimozide	Orap®	Neuroleptic	Tourette
Pioglitazone	Actos®	Thiazolidinedione	Diabetes
Pirbuterol	Maxair®	Inhaled Bronchodilator	Asthma
Piroxicam	Feldene®	NSAID	Lupus
Podofilox	Condylox®	Antimitotic	STD
Podophyllin	Podofin®	Antimitotic	STD
Prednisolone	Prelone®	Corticosteroid	Asthma; Eczema
Prednisone	Deltasone®	Corticosteroid	JRA; Asthma; Allergies; Eczema; IBS; Kidney Disease; Lupus

Generic Name	Brand Name	Category	Use
Primidone	Mysoline®	Anticonvulsant	Seizures
Prochlorperazine	Compazine®	Antinausea	Migraine
Promethazine	Phenergan®	Antinausea	Migraine
Propoxyphene/ Acetaminophen	Darvocet-N®	Analgesic/Narcotic	Migraine
Propoxyphene/Aspirin/ Caffeine	Darvon Compound®	Analgesic/Narcotic	Migraine
Propranolol	Inderal®	Beta-Blocker	Anxiety; Migraine
Protriptyline	Vivactil®	Tricyclic Antidepressant	Migraine
Pseudoephedrine	Sudafed®	Decongestant OTC	Allergies
Pyrethrins/ Piperonyl Butoxide	Rid®	Pediculocide	STD
Resorcinol	Acnomel®	OTC Acne Medication	Acne
Risperidone	Risperdal®	Neuroleptic	Tourette
Ritonavir	Norvir®	Protease Inhibitor	STD
Rizatriptan	Maxalt®	Triptan	Migraine
Rosiglitazone	Avandia®	Thiazolidinedione	Diabetes
Salicylic Acid	Oxy Clean®	OTC Acne Medication	Acne
Salmeterol	Serevent®	Inhaled Bronchodilator	Asthma

Salmeterol and Fluticasone	Advair Diskus®	Inhaled Bronchodilator	Asthma
Saquinavir	Fortovase®	Protease Inhibitor	STD
Sertraline	Zoloft®	SSRI	Anxiety; Depression; Eating Disorders; Migraine
Spironolactone	Aldactone®	Diuretic	Kidney Disease
Stavudine	Zerit®	NRTI	STD
Sulfasalazine	Azulfidine®	Aminosalicylate	DMARD; IBD; JRA
Sulfur	Cuticura®	OTC Acne Medication	Acne
Sulindac	Clinoril®	NSAID	Lupus
Sumatriptan	Imitrex®	Triptan	Migraine
Tacrolimus	Protopic®	Topical Immunomodulator	Eczema
Tazarotene	Tazorac®	Topical Retinoid	Acne
Tetracycline	Achromycin V®	Antibiotic	Acne; STD
Tetrahydrozoline	Tyzine®	Decongestant Nasal Spray	Allergies
Theophylline	Elixophyllin®	Systemic Bronchodilator	Asthma
Tiagabine	Gabitril®	Mood Stabilizer/Anticonvulsant	Depression; Seizures; Migraine
Topiramate	Topamax®	Mood Stabilizer/Anticonvulsant	Depression; Migraine; Seizures

Generic	Brand	Class	Condition
Torsemide	Demadex®	Diuretic	Kidney Disease
Tramadol/Acetaminophen	Ultracet®	Analgesic	JRA
Tranylcypromine	Parnate®	MAOI	Anxiety
Trazodone	Desyrel®	Atypical Antidepressants	Anxiety; Depression
Tretinoin	Retin-A®	Topical Retinoid	Acne
Triamcinolone	Aristocort®	Corticosteroid	Asthma
Triamcinolone	Aristocort®	Topical Corticosteroid	Eczema; Lupus
Triamcinolone	Azmacort®	Corticosteroid—Inhaled	Asthma
Triamcinolone	Nasacort®	Corticosteroid—Nasal Spray	Allergies
Triamterene	Dyrenium®	Diuretic	Kidney Disease
Trichloroacetic Acid	TCA®	Topical Acid	STD
Trolamine Salicylate	Aspercreme®	Topical Analgesic	JRA
Ultralente Insulin	Humulin U®	Long-acting Insulin	Diabetes
Valacyclovir	Valtrex®	Antiviral	STDs
Valdecoxib	Bextra®	COX-2 Inhibitor/NSAID	JRA
Valproic Acid	Depakene®	Mood Stabilizer/Anticonvulsant	Anxiety; Depression; Seizures
Venlafaxine	Effexor®	Atypical Antidepressants	Anxiety; Depression
Verapamil	Isoptin®	Calcium Channel Blocker	Migraine

Zafirlukast	Accolate®	Leukotriene Modifier	Allergies; Asthma
Zalcitabine	Hivid®	NRTI	STD
Zidovudine (AZT)	Retrovir®	NRTI	STD
Zileuton	Zyflo®	Leukotriene Modifier	Allergies; Asthma
Zolmitriptan	Zomig®	Triptan	Migraine
Zonisamide	Zonegran®	Anticonvulsant	Seizures

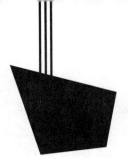

Medication Diary

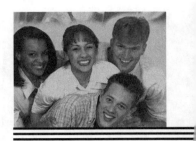

Medical Information

Primary Doctor:_____ Phone:_____

Specialist:_____ Phone:_____

Contact in an Emergency:_____ Phone:_____

Pharmacy:_____ Phone:_____

Medication Information

Name of Medication:_____

Date Begun:_____

Dosage:_____

Special Instructions:_____

Listing of Side Effects:

Date/Time	Dosage	Reactions	Notes

Medication Information

Name of Medication: _____

Date Begun: _____

Dosage: _____

Special Instructions: _____

Listing of Side Effects:

Date/Time	Dosage	Reactions	Notes

Medication Information

Name of Over-the-Counter Medication: _____

Date Begun: _____

Dosage: _____

Special Instructions: _____

Listing of Side Effects:

Date/Time	Dosage	Reactions	Notes

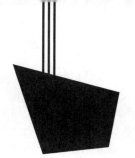

Bibliography

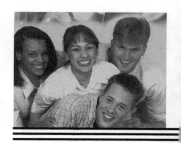

GENERAL

Azarnoff, Pat. *Health, Illness and Disability: A Guide to Books for Children and Young Adults*. New York: R.R. Bowker Company, 1983.

Buchman, Dian Dincin. *Ancient Healing Secrets*. New York: Crescent Books, 1996.

Burger, Alfred. *Drugs and People, Medications, Their History and Origins, and the Way They Act*. Charlottesville: University Press of Virginia, 1986.

"Drug Information." U.S. National Library of Medicine and National Institutes of Health, 2003, at www.nlm.nih.gov/medlineplus/druginformation.html (last accessed 11 November 2003).

"Drug Search." Mayo Foundation for Medical Education and Research, 2003, at www.mayoclinic.com/findinformation/ druginformation/index.cfm (last accessed 11 November 2003).

"Drugs." WholeHealthMD.com, 2000, at www.wholehealth md.com/refshelf/drugs_index/1,1521,,00.html (last accessed 11 November 2003).

Elliott, Victoria Stagg. "Study Suggests Link Between NSAIDs, Aspirin, Miscarriage." *American Medical News*, 6 October 2003, at www.ama-assn.org/amednews/ 2003/10/06/hlse1006.htm (last accessed 11 November 2003).

Bibliography

Farley, Dixie. "Benefit Vs. Risk: How FDA Approves New Drugs." *FDA Consumer Special Report*, January 1995, at www.fda.gov/fdac/special/newdrug/benefits.html (last accessed 24 November 2003).

Griffith, H. Winter. *Complete Guide to Prescription and Nonprescription Drugs, Edition 2002*. New York: Berkley Publishing Group, 2001.

Kaufman, Miriam. *Easy for You to Say: Q & As for Teens Living with Chronic Illness or Disability*. Toronto: Key Porter Books Limited, 1995.

LeVert, Suzanne, and Julian Messner. *Teens Face to Face with Chronic Illness*. New York: Simon & Schuster, 1993.

Levine, Milton I., and Jean H. Seligmann. *The Parents' Encyclopedia of Infancy, Childhood and Adolescence*. New York: Thomas Y. Crowell Company, 1973.

"Medication Index." MedicineNet.com, 2003, at www.medicine net.com/medications/article.htm (last accessed 11 November 2003).

Nickel, Robert E., and Larry W. Desch, eds. *The Physician's Guide to Caring for Children with Disabilities and Chronic Conditions*. Baltimore, Md.: Paul H. Brookes Publishing Co., Inc., 2000.

Paquette, Penny Hutchins, and Cheryl Gerson Tuttle. *Parenting a Child with a Behavior Problem*. Los Angeles: Lowell House, 1999.

Porter, Roy, ed.. *The Cambridge Illustrated History of Medicine*. Cambridge: Cambridge University Press, 1966.

"Prescription Drugs and Pain Medications." National Institute on Drug Abuse, Research Report Series: Prescription Drugs/Abuse and Addiction, April 2001, at www.nida.nih.gov/Infofax/PainMed.html (last accessed 10 November 2003).

Rybacki, James, *The Essential Guide to Prescription Drugs 2002*. New York: Harper Resource, 2001.

Silverman, Harold M., ed. *The Pill Book*. New York: Bantam Books, 2002.

Wilens, Timothy E. *Straight Talk about Psychiatric Medications for Kids*. New York: Guilford Press, 1999.

202

ACNE

"Acne." National Library of Medicine, 2002, at www.nlm.nih.gov/medlineplus/tutorials/acne/dm019101 .html (last accessed 3 September 2003).

"Acne Myths." Acne Net, American Academy of Dermatology, 2002, at www.skincarephysicians.com/ acnenet/myths.html (last accessed 26 February 2003).

"Acne Treatments." Acne.com, 2003–2003, at www.healthplug .com/acne_treatments.html (last accessed 1 March 2003).

"Combination Therapies Offer New Management Options of Acne and Rosacea." American Academy of Dermatology, 17 October 2001, at www.aad.org/PressReleases/ combination.html (last accessed 26 February 2003).

"The Lowdown on Blackheads." Acne Net, American Academy of Dermatology, 2002, at www.skincare physicians.com/acnenet/update.html (last accessed 26 February 2003).

"Medical and Aesthetic Lasers." Candela, 2002, at www .candelalaser.com (last accessed 26 February 2003).

"Oral Contraceptives and Acne." The Aware Foundation, 2003, at www.awarefoundation.org/aware/articles/ oral_contraceptives.asp (last accessed 26 February 2003).

"Over-the-Counter Products." Acne Net, American Academy of Dermatology, 2002 at www.skincarephysicians.com/ acnenet/overthecounter.html (last accessed 26 February 2003).

"Prescription Medications." Acne Net, American Academy of Dermatology, 2002, at www.skincarephysicians.com/ acnenet/precriptmeds.html (last accessed 20 August 2002).

Questions and Answers about Acne. Bethesda, Md.: National Institute of Arthritis and Musculoskeletal and Skin Diseases (NIAMS), National Institute of Health, Public Health Service, U.S. Department of Public Health, NIH Publication No. 01-4998, October 2001.

"The Role of a Physician." Acne Net, American Academy of Dermatology, 2002, at www.skincarephysicians.com/ acnenet/treatmnt.html (last accessed 5 November 2002).

"Treating Acne." American Academy of Pediatrics, 2000, at www.medem.com/search/article_display.cfm?path=\\ TANQUERAY\M_ContentItem&mstr=/M_ContentItem/ ZZZKRFFGL5C.html&soc=AAP&srch_typ=NAV_ SERCH (last accessed 26 February 2003).

ADHD

"Atomoxetine HCI." Stratera, Atomoxetine HCI Pharmacology—ADHD Medication, 2002, at www .healthyplace.com/medications/strattera.htm (last accessed 27 February 2003).

"Medical Management of Children and Adults with AD/HD." *Children and Adults with Attention-Deficit Hyperactivity Disorder Fact Sheet #3*, 2000, at www.chadd.org/fs/fs3.htm.

Michelson, David, Douglas Faries, Joachim Wernicke, Douglas Kelsey, Katherine Kendrick, F. Randy Sallee, Thomas Spencer, and the Atomoxetine ADHD Study Group. "Atomoxetine in the Treatment of Children and Adolescents with Attention-Deficit/Hyperactivity Disorder: A Randomized, Placebo-Controlled, Dose-Response Study." *Pediatrics* 108, no. 5 (November 5, 2001), e83, at www.pediatrics.org/cgi/content/full/108/5/e83 (last accessed 6 September 2002).

National Institute on Drug Abuse. *The Brain & the Actions of Cocaine, Opiates, and Marijuana—Slide Teaching Packet for Scientists.* Washington, DC: U.S. Department of Health and Human Services, National Institutes of Health, 2003.

Neuwirth, Sharyn M. *Attention Deficit Hyperactivity Disorder.* National Institutes of Health, Publication No. 96-3572, 1996, at www.nimh.nih.gov/publicat/adhd.cfm (last accessed 27 February 2003).

Silver, Dr. Larry. "Update on ADHD Medications." *Learning Disabilities OnLine*, May 2002, at www.ldonline.org/ ld_indepth/add_adhd/adhd_medications_update.html (last accessed 27 February 2003).

Spencer, T., and J. Biederman. "Non-stimulant Treatment for Attention-Deficit/Hyperactivity Disorder." *Journal of Attention Disorders*, 6, suppl. 1 (2002), 109–114.

Wilens, Timothy E., and Thomas J. Spencer. "The Stimulants Revisited." *Child and Adolescent Psychiatric Clinics of North America*, 9, no. 3 (July 2000), 573–594.

ALLERGIES

"Fast Facts: Allergies." American Academy of Allergy, Asthma and Immunology, 2002, at www.aaaai.org/patients/resources/fastfacts/allergies.stm (last accessed 17 August 2003).

Geimeier, William. "Nut and Peanut Allergy." The Nemours Foundation, 2003, at www.kidshealth.org/parent/growth/feeding/nut_peanut_allergy.html (last accessed 3 November 2003).

"Medications for Allergies." Mayo Foundation for Medical Education and Research, 2003, at www.mayoclinic.com/findinformation/conditioncenters/subcenters.cfm?objectid=66F15D74-DE7A-433F-8E29447C3A7648A4 (last accessed 3 December 2002).

"Tips to Remember: What is an Allergic Reaction." American Academy of Allergy, Asthma and Immunology, 2003, at www.aaaai.org/patients/publicedmat/tips/whatisallergic reaction.stm (last accessed 17 August 2003).

ANXIETY

Anxiety Disorders. National Institutes of Health, Publication No. 02-3879, 1994, 1995/2000/2002, at www.nimh.nih.gov/anxiety/anxiety.cfm (last accessed 7 August 2003).

Anxiety Disorders Research at the National Institute of Mental Health. National Institutes of Health, Publication No. 99-4504, 1999, at www.nimh.nih.gov/publicat/anxresfact.cfm (last accessed 7 August 2003).

Facts about Anxiety Disorders. National Institute of Mental Health, Publication No. OM-994152, January 1999/April

2003, at www.nimh.nih.gov/anxiety/adfacts.cfm (last accessed 7 August 2003).

"Medications." Anxiety Disorders Association of America, 2003, at www.adaa.org/AnxietyDisorderInfor/ Medications.cfm (last accessed 7 August 2003).

Morton, W. Alexander. "Anxiety Disorders: Treatment and Counseling." *U.S. Pharmacist*, October 2002, at www.uspharmacist.com/index.asp?page=ce/anxiety_ treatment/default.htm (last accessed 7 August 2003).

Sajatovic, Martha. "Treatment for Mood and Anxiety Disorders: Quetiapine and Aripiprazole." Department of Psychiatry, Case Western Reserve University, 2003, at www.docguide. com/news/content.nsf/PaperFrameSet?OpenForm&newsid= 8525697700573E1885256D6500322861&topabstract= 1&u=http://www.ncbi.nlm.nih.gov/entrez/query.fcgi?cmd= Retrieve&db=PubMed&dopt=Abstract&list_uids=128575 36 (last accessed 15 August 2003).

ASTHMA

"Asthma in Children Fact Sheet." American Lung Association, March 2003, at www.lungusa.org/asthma/ascpedfac99 .html (last accessed 7 September 2003).

Hannaway, Dr. Paul J. *Asthma—An Emerging Epidemic*. Marblehead, Mass.: Lighthouse Press, 2002.

Hogan, Martha, Neil MacIntyre, Michael Mellon, and Dennis Williams. "Noisy and Quiet Asthma Medication." *Allergy & Asthma Health Consumer Guide 2003*, at www.aanma.org/pharmacy/ph_med_asthmamed.htm (last accessed 29 September 2003).

Mayo Clinic Staff. "Medications and Immunotherapy for Asthma." Mayo Foundation for Medical Education and Research, October 28, 2003, at www.mayoclinic.com/invoke.cfm?id=AP00008 (last accessed 9 September 2003).

Meadows, Michelle. "Breathing Better: Action Plans Keep Asthma in Check." FDA Consumer Magazine (March–April 2003).

Paquette, Penny Hutchins. *Asthma: The Ultimate Teen Guide*. Lanham, Md.: Scarecrow Press, 2003.

Rutherford, Kim. "Asthma." Teens Health, The Nemours Foundation, May 2001, at kidshealth.org/PageManager. jsp?dn=KidsHealth&lic=1&ps=207&cat_id=20168& article_set=20581 (last accessed 7 September 2003).

"Students with Chronic Illnesses: Guidance for Families, Schools and Students." National Heart, Lung and Blood Institute, 2003, at www.nhlbi.nih.gov/health/public/lung/ asthma/guidfam.htm (last accessed 7 September 2003).

"Tips to Remember: Childhood Asthma." American Academy of Allergy, Asthma & Immunology, 2003, at www.aaaai.org/patients/publicedmat/tips/childhoodasth- ma.stm (last accessed 7 September 2003).

"What Is Asthma." Asthma and Allergy Foundation of America, 2003, at www.aafa.org/templ/display.cfm?id= 2&sub=25 (last accessed 29 September 2003).

DEPRESSION

Ascher, J. A., J. O. Cole, J. N. Colin, J. P. Feighner, R. M. Ferris, H. C. Fibiger, R. N. Golden, P. Martin, W. Z. Potter, E. Richelson, et al. Department of Neurology/Psychiatry, Burroughs Wellcome Co. "Bupropion: A Review of Its Mechanism of Antidepressant Activity." *Journal of Clinical Psychiatry,* 56, no. 9 (September 1995): 395–401.

Cox, David E. "Common Pharmacological Treatments of Bipolar Disorder and Subtypes: A Review." Florida Gulf Coast University, April 1999, at itech.fgcu.edu/&/issues/ vol2/issue1/bipolar.htm (last accessed 4 August 2003).

DeJong, Sandra. "An Introduction to Pediatric Psychopharmacology." Emotional Health for Children: Parents and Doctors as Partners, December 2002, at www.drkingsoffice.com/GS_psychopharm.html (last accessed 4 September 2003).

Depression. National Institutes of Health, Publication No. 02- 3561, 2002, at www.nimh.nih.gov/publicat/depression .cfm (last accessed 1 August 2003).

Lutz, Katherine. "Can a Popular Antidepressant Cause Teenage Suicide?" *The Boston Globe* (5 August 2003), pp. D1,4.

Lyness, D'Arcy. "Types of Depression." The Nemours Foundation, at kidshealth.org/teen/your_mind/mental_health/depression_p3.html (last accessed 4 August 2003).

Medications. National Institutes of Health, Publication No. 02-3929, 2002, at www.nimh.nih.gov/publicat/medicate.cfm (last accessed 4 August 2003).

"Now We Can Successfully Treat the Illness Called Depression." National Foundation for Depressive Illness, Inc., 2003, at www.depression.org, (last accessed 4 August 2003).

DIABETES

"Diabetes Pills." U.S. Food and Drug Administration, 2002, at www.fda.gov/diabetes/pills.html (last accessed 1 May 2002).

"Diabetes: Why You Need Insulin and How to Use It." American Academy of Family Physicians, 2001, at familydoctor.org/handouts/354.html (last accessed 31 July 2003).

Dowshen, Steve. "Insulin-Dependant Diabetes." The Nemours Foundation, July 2001, at kidshealth.org/parent/medical/endocrine/diabetes_p5.html (last accessed 31 July 2003).

"Helping the Student with Diabetes Succeed, A Guide for School Personnel." U.S. Department of Health and Human Services, June 2003, at ndep.nih.gov/materials/pubs/schoolguide.pdf (last accessed 31 July 2003).

"Insulin Preparations." U.S. Food and Drug Administration, *FDA Consumer Magazine*, January–February 2002, at www.fda.gov/fdac/features/2002/chrt_insulin.html (last accessed 31 July 2003).

Lewis, Carol. "Diabetes: A Growing Public Health Concern." U.S. Food and Drug Administration, *FDA Consumer Magazine*, January–February 2002, at www.fda.gov/fdac/features/2002/102_diab.html (last accessed 31 July 2003).

Medicines for People with Diabetes. National Institutes of Health, Publication No. 03-4222, December 2002, at diabetes.niddk.nih.gov/dm/pubs/medicines_ez/index .htm#6 (last accessed 31 July 2003).

"Oral Antidiabetes Medications." U.S. Food and Drug Administration, *FDA Consumer Magazine*, January–February 2002, at www.fda.gov/fdac/features/ 2002/chrt_oralmeds.html (last accessed 31 July 2003).

"Quick Information—Diabetes." U.S. Food and Drug Administration, 2002, at www.fda.gov/opacom/lowlit/ diabetes.html (last accessed 31 July 2003).

Saudek, Christopher D., Richard R. Rubin, and Cynthia S. Shump. *The Johns Hopkins Guide to Diabetes*. Baltimore: Johns Hopkins University Press, 1997.

EATING DISORDERS

Eating Disorders: Facts about Eating Disorders and the Search for Solutions. National Institutes of Health, Publication No. 01-4901, 2001, at www.nimh.nih.gov/ publicat/eatingdisorder.cfm (last accessed 12 April 2003).

Rutherford, Kim. "Eating Disorders: Anorexia and Bulimia." The Nemours Foundation, September 2001, at www .kidshealth.org/teen/your_mind/mental_health/eat_ disorder.html (last accessed 6 August 2003).

ECZEMA

"Eczema: Frequently Asked Questions." National Eczema Society, 2003, at www.eczema.org, (last accessed 11 August 2003).

Corssen, Dr. John, Jon Hanifin, Amy Paller, Hugh Sampson, and Mary Spraker. "Atopic Dermatitis in Children." The National Eczema Association for Science and Education, 2003, at www.nationaleczema.org (last accessed 11 August 2003).

Dowshen, Steve. "All about Eczema." The Nemours Foundation, August 2003, at kidshealth.org/teen/

diseases_conditions/allergies_immune/eczema.html (last accessed 11 August 2003).

Handout on Health: Atopic Dermatitis. National Institute of Arthritis and Musculoskeletal and Skin Diseases, National Institutes of Health, Publication No. 03-4272, April 2003, at www.niams.nih.gov/hi/topics/dermatitis/ index.html (last accessed 11 August 2003).

"Eczema Treatment." American Academy of Dermatology, 2000 at www.skincarephysicians.com/eczemanet/treatment .html (last accessed 11 August 2003).

"EczemaNet Update: Treating Eczema with Steroids." American Academy of Dermatology, 2000, at www .skincarephysicians.com/eczemanet/update_current.html (last accessed 11 August 2003).

INFLAMMATORY BOWEL DISEASE

Dallek, Robert. *An Unfinished Life, John F. Kennedy 1917–1963.* Boston: Little Brown and Company, 2003.

"Introduction to Crohn's Disease." Crohn's and Colitis Foundation of America, 2003, at www.ccfa.org/medinfo/ medinfo/aboutcd.html (last accessed 21 August 2003).

"Introduction to Ulcerative Colitis." Crohn's and Colitis Foundation of America, 2003, at www.ccfa.org/medinfo/ medinfo/aboutuc.html (last accessed 21 August 2003).

Kam, Lori, and Jay W. Marks, eds. "Crohn's Disease." MedicineNet, Inc. February 2002, at www.medicinenet .com/Crohns_Disease/article.htm (last accessed 21 August 2003).

Shaffer, Stephen. "Inflammatory Bowel Disease." The Nemours Foundation, February 2001, at kidshealth.org/ teen/diseases_conditions/digestive/ibd.html (last accessed 21 August 2003).

JUVENILE RHEUMATOID ARTHRITIS

Arthritis in Children. Bethesda, Md.: National Institute of Arthritis and Musculoskeletal and Skin Diseases, National Institutes of Health, January 2000.

Dunkin, Mary Anne. "2003 Drug Guide." *Arthritis Today*, 2003.

"Juvenile Arthritis." American College of Rheumatology, September 2003, at www.rheumatology.org/patients/factsheet/jra.html (last accessed 10 November 2003).

"Juvenile Rheumatoid Arthritis." American Academy of Orthopaedic Surgeons, July 2001, at orthoinfo.aaos.org/fact/thr_report.cfm?Thread_ID=303&topcategory=Arthritis (last accessed 30 July 2003).

Progress & Promise. Bethesda, Md.: National Institute of Arthritis and Musculoskeletal and Skin Diseases, National Institutes of Health, Publication No. 01-4939, March 2001.

Rheumatoid Arthritis. Bethesda, Md.: National Institute of Arthritis and Musculoskeletal and Skin Diseases, National Institutes of Health, Publication No. 00-4179, November 1999.

"School Success." Arthritis Foundation, 2003, at www.arthritis.org/resources/school_success.asp (last accessed 30 July 2003).

Serrate-Sztein, Susana, Lauren Pachman, Patience White, Edward H. Giannini, and David Glass. *Questions and Answers about Juvenile Rheumatoid Arthritis*. Bethesda, Md.: National Institute of Arthritis and Musculoskeletal and Skin Diseases, National Institutes of Health, Publication No. 01-4942, July 2001, at www.niams.nih.gov/hi/topics/juvenile_arthritis/juvarthr.htm (last accessed 30 July 2003).

KIDNEY CONDITIONS

Amtmann-Buettner, Kim. *Kidney Beginnings: A Patient's Guide to Living with Reduced Kidney Function*. Tampa, Fla.: American Association of Kidney Patients, 2003.

"Diuretics." Altruis Biomedical Network, 2002, at www.e-kidneys.net/diuretics.html (last accessed 27 August 2003).

Hopp, Laszlo. "Chronic Kidney Conditions." The Nemours Foundation, April 2001, at kidshealth.org/teen/diseases_conditions/urinary/kidney.html (last accessed 27 August 2003).

Hopp, Laszlo. "When Your Child Has a Chronic Kidney Disease." The Nemours Foundation, May 2001, at

www.kidshealth.org/parent/medical/kidney/chronic_
kidney_disease.html (last accessed 3 November 2003).

Ogbru, Omudhome, and Jay Marks, eds. "Calcium Channel
Blockers (CCBs)." MedicineNet, Inc., April 2002, at
www.medicinenet.com/Calcium_Channel_Blockers/article
.htm (last accessed 27 August 2003).

LUPUS

Aranow, Cynthia, and Arthur Weinstein. "Non-Steroidal Anti-
Inflammatory Drugs (NSAIDs)." Lupus Foundation of
America, 2001, at www.lupus.org/education/brochures/
nsaid.html (last accessed 22 August 2003).

Dowshen, Steve. "Life with Lupus." The Nemours
Foundation, March 2001, at kidshealth.org/teen/
diseases_conditions/bones/lupus.html (last accessed 22
August 2003).

Gluck, Oscar. "Anti-Malarials in the Treatment of Lupus."
Lupus Foundation of America, 2000, at www.lupus
.org/education/brochures/antimalarials01.html (last
accessed 22 August 2003).

Katz, Robert S. "Immune Suppressants and Related Drugs
Used for Lupus." Lupus Foundation of America, Inc.,
2001, at www.lupus.org/education/brochures/immune
.html (last accessed 22 August 2003).

Klippel, John 'Jack' H. "Medications." Lupus Foundation of
America, Inc., 2001, at www.lupus.org/education/
brochures/medications.html (last accessed 22 August 2003).

Systemic Lupus Erythematosus. Bethesda, Md.: National
Institute of Arthritis and Musculoskeletal and Skin
Diseases, National Institutes of Health, Publication No.
97-4178, February 2000, at www.niams.nih.gov/hi/
topics/lupus/slehandout/index.htm#Lupus_6 (last
accessed 22 August 2003).

MIGRAINE

"Children and Migraines" American Medical Association,
1998, at www.medem.com/medlb/article_detaillb.cfm?

article_ID=ZZZIAZF99CC&sub_cat=567 (last accessed 9 October 2003).

"Drugs for Mild-to-Moderate Migraine and Tension-Type Headache Pain." American Medical Association, 1998, at www.medem.com/medlb/article_detaillb.cfm?article_ID=ZZZDZ91PACC&sub_cat=567 (last accessed 9 October 2003).

"Drugs That Prevent Migraine." American Medical Association, 1998, at www.medem.com/medlb/article_detaillb.cfm?article_ID=ZZZYCRLPACC&sub_cat=567 (last accessed 9 October 2003).

"How is Migraine Treated." American Medical Association, 1998, at www.medem.com/medlb/article_detaillb.cfm?article_ID=ZZZ671XPACC&sub_cat=567 (last accessed 9 October 2003).

Klapper, Jack A. "Botox and Migraine." *Headache*, the Newsletter of American Council for Headache Education, 12, no. 1 (Spring 2001), at www.achenet.org/articles/24.php (last accessed 9 October 2003).

"Migraines in Children and Adolescents." The Cleveland Clinic, 2003, at www.clevelandclinic.org/health/health-info/docs/2500/2555.asp?index=9637 (last accessed 9 October 2003).

Rust, Robert S. "Treatment of Pediatric Migraine." Practical Neurology, at www.healthsystem.virginia.edu/internet/neurogram/neurogram3_4_peds_migraines.cfm (last accessed 9 October 2003).

SEXUALLY TRANSMITTED DISEASES

"Common Antibiotics." Alliance for the Prudent Use of Antibiotics, 2002, at www.tufts.edu/med/apua/Miscellaneous/common_antibiotics.html (last accessed 26 August 2003).

"Fact Sheet: New CDC Treatment Guidelines Critical to Preventing Health Consequences of Sexually Transmitted Diseases." United States Department of Health and Human Services, Centers for Disease

213

Control and Prevention, May 2002, at www.cdc.gov/od/oc/media/pressrel/fs020509.htm (last accessed 26 August 2003).

"Information to Live By: Chlamydia." American Social Health Association, 2001, at www.ashastd.org/stdfaqs/chlamydia.html (last accessed 25 August 2003).

"Information to Live By: Crabs." American Social Health Association, 2001, at www.ashastd.org/stdfaqs/crabs.html (last accessed 25 August 2003).

"Information to Live By: Gonorrhea." American Social Health Association, 2001, at www.ashastd.org/stdfaqs/gonorrhea.html (last accessed 25 August 2003).

Mayo Clinic Staff. "Chlamydia: Treatment." Mayo Foundation for Medical Information and Research, August 2003, at www.mayoclinic.com/invoke.cfm?objectid=76877F15-F95F-44BB85C8B47F756CBA49&section=7 (last accessed 25 August 2003).

Mayo Clinic Staff. "Genital Herpes: Treatment." Mayo Foundation for Medical Information and Research, August 2003, at www.mayoclinic.com/invoke.cfm?objectid=345386D6-9612-409A-9D87D869D4913E44&section=6 (last accessed 25 August 2003).

Mayo Clinic Staff. "Genital Warts: Treatment, Mayo Foundation for Medical Information and Research, June 2003, at www.mayoclinic.com/invoke.cfm?objectid=CAEC99AC-77E1-414C-B0A8ACFA312F2E1E&section=7 (last accessed 25 August 2003).

"Sexually Transmitted Diseases." Patient Education Institute, Medline Plus, October 2001, at www.nlm.nih.gov/medlineplus/tutorials/sexuallytransmitteddiseases/hp079101.html (last accessed 26 August 2003).

"STDs: Common Symptoms & Tips on Prevention." American Academy of Family Physicians Family Health Facts, July 2003, at familydoctor.org/healthfacts/165/ (last accessed 26 August 2003).

"T-20 (Enfuvirtide)." Project Inform, October 2003, at www.projinf.org/fs/enfuvirtide.html (last accessed 2 November 2003).

SEIZURES

"Epilepsy and Seizures: Hope Through Research." National Institute of Neurological Disorders and Stroke, National Institutes of Health, April 2000, at www.medem.com/search/article_display.cfm?path=\\TANQUERAY\M_ContentItem&mstr=/M_ContentItem/ZZZF4GBUU7C.html&soc=NIH&srch_typ=NAV_SERCH (last accessed 9 October 2003).

"Epilepsy/Seizures: Treatment." Health Communities.com, 2003, at www.neurologychannel.com/seizures/treatment.shtml (last accessed 9 October 2003).

"What is Epilepsy." National Institute of Neurological Disorders and Stroke, National Institutes of Health, August 2000, at www.medem.com/search/article_display.cfm?path=\\TANQUERAY\M_ContentItem&mstr=/M_ContentItem/ZZZIV7SJ7JC.html&soc=NIH&srch_typ=NAV_SERCH (last accessed 9 October 2003).

TOURETTE SYNDROME

Bartnett, Joy E., and Joseph Jankovic. "Tourette's Syndrome: Information for Patients and Caregivers." Worldwide Education and Awareness for Movement Disorders, August 2003, at www.wemove.org/ts/default.htm (last accessed 13 August 2003).

Gay, Kathlyn, and Sean McGarrahan. *Epilepsy: The Ultimate Teen Guide*. Lanham, Md.: Scarecrow Press, 2003.

Kurlan, Roger. "Medications and Dosages, Current Pharmacology of Tourette Syndrome." Tourette Syndrome Association, Inc., 2002, at tsa-usa.org/ (last accessed 13 August 2003).

"Tourette Syndrome Fact Sheet." National Institute of Neurological Disorders and Stroke, Tourette Syndrome Association, July 2001, at www.ninds.nih.gov/health_and_medical/pubs/tourette_syndrome.htm#whatis (last accessed 13 August 2003).

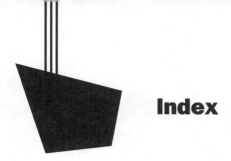

Index

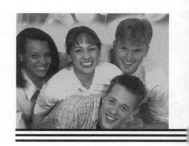

Italics denote sidebars.

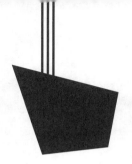

About the Author

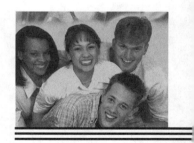

Cheryl Gerson Tuttle has more than thirty years of experience in education, counseling, and advocacy. She is coauthor of five other books: *Thinking Games to Play with Your Child: Easy Ways to Develop Creative and Critical Thinking Skills* (1991, 1997), *Parenting a Child with a Learning Disability* (1995), *Challenging Voices: Writings by, for, and about Individuals with Learning Disabilities* (1995), *Parenting a Child with a Behavior Problem: A Practical and Empathetic Guide* (1999), and *Learning Disabilities: The Ultimate Teen Guide* (Scarecrow, 2003).